OVERCOMING
THE THREAT
OF DEATH

Overcoming the Threat of Death

A Journal of One Christian's Encounter with Cancer

ARIE BROUWER

WILLIAM B. EERDMANS PUBLISHING COMPANY
GRAND RAPIDS, MICHIGAN

© 1994 WCC Publications
World Council of Churches
Geneva, Switzerland

This edition published 1994 through special
arrangement with WCC Publications by
Wm. B. Eerdmans Publishing Co.
255 Jefferson Ave. S.E., Grand Rapids, Michigan 49503
Printed in the United States of America

00 99 98 97 96 95 94   7 6 5 4 3 2 1

Library of Congress Cataloging-in-Publication Data

Brouwer, Arie R.
    Overcoming the threat of death: a journal of one Christian's
encounter with cancer / Arie Brouwer.
        p.   cm.
    ISBN 0-8028-0833-6 (pbk.)
    1. Cancer — Patients — Religious life. 2. Brouwer, Arie R.
3. Cancer — Patients — Biography. 4. Ecumenical movement.
5. Christian life — Reformed Church authors.   I. Title.
BV4910.33.B76   1994
248.8′6 — dc20   94-3387
                                                        CIP

For Harriet

who has walked with me through it all
and whose love daily astonishes me
while filling me with wonder and thanksgiving

There can hardly be a better image of caring than that of the artist who brings new life to people by an honest and fearless self-portrait. Rembrandt painted his sixty-three self-portraits not just as "a model for studies in expression" but as "a search for the spiritual through the channel of his innermost personality"...

Rembrandt realized that what is most personal is most universal. We are able really to care only if we are willing to paint and repaint constantly our self-portrait, not as a morbid self-preoccupation, but as a service to those who are searching for some light in the midst of the darkness.

To care one must offer one's own vulnerable self to others as a source of healing...

Henri Nouwen
Aging
(emphasis added)

Table of Contents

ix   FOREWORD

1   1. DISCOVERING A MALIGNANT TUMOR

7   2. SETTLING INTO THE STRUGGLE

13   3. DECIDING ABOUT SURGERY AND CHEMOTHERAPY

19   4. WHY?

25   5. THE RELATIVITY OF TIME AND THE
        TRANSFIGURATION OF THE WORLD

31   6. THE FUNERAL AS FINAL OFFERING

46   7. FORMS OF SUPPORT

53   8. UNFINISHED BUSINESS — PERSONAL
        RELATIONSHIPS

59   9. UNFINISHED BUSINESS — MY ECUMENICAL
        VOCATION

70   10. HEALING AND FAITH

80   POSTSCRIPT — GROWING IN GRACE

        APPENDIXES

84   1. "I AM THE WAY, THE TRUTH AND THE LIFE"

93   2. "I BELIEVE IN THE COMMUNION OF SAINTS"

100   3. SOME NOTES ON ECUMENICAL IMMOBILITY

Foreword

The reflections that constitute this small volume emerged first in the form of therapy. Although I have never consistently kept a journal, through most of my professional life writing has been a major means of clarifying what I think and of sorting out what I feel. At no time have I felt a greater need for such clarifying and sorting than in the past few months since I was diagnosed as having cancer.

Almost immediately, I found that these reflections were a useful way to inform friends and family, most of whom live at considerable distances from us. Retelling the story of my cancer over and over on the telephone, I found depressing, whereas saying it once in writing and sending the story around helped to clear it up for me, and to give people some guidance as to how they could best support me and my family.

Already by the second reflection I knew that I was writing as well for the Community Church at Glen Rock. I had been serving that congregation for only about ten weeks as interim pastor, but Harriet and I were long-time (25 years) members, though somewhat irregular in attendance, because my work often took me elsewhere on Sunday. It was fertile soil for the rapid development of deeply meaningful relationships. I wanted to stay in touch — and they wanted me to.

The feedback from family, friends and the congregation was instant and overwhelming. Many wrote or called to say how helpful the reflections had been to them personally and in many cases that they had passed them along to others whom they were sure would also benefit from them. Many urged that the reflections be published.

Some friends at the World Council of Churches, Wesley and Karin Granberg-Michaelson, went further and actually proposed that the World Council of Churches publish them. The Council seemed eager to do so. That news came to me between journal entries 5 and 6, when there had already been a hiatus of almost four months because I was devoting all the energy I had for writing to sermons.

By the time I started writing these journal entries again I had also been forced by lack of strength and energy to give up my interim pastoral duties. That relentless advance of the disease put me in a different place from where I was while writing the first five reflections — a place of recognition that death was probably not far off. I wanted therefore not only to reflect on my present experiences but past ones as well, to try in at least some sketchy fashion to "wrap it all up".

These two factors, the knowledge that I was writing for publication and the desire to see the picture whole, gave a different quality to some of the last five reflections. The fact that the World Council would be the publisher was also important. That left me free to reflect on my ecumenical vocation. With another publisher, such reflection might have seemed an intrusion. My friends at the World Council of Churches would know better. They would know that without such reflection this volume would be seriously incomplete, since the ecumenical movement has been at the centre of my life for at least the last twenty-five years.

Nevertheless, in spite of these differences between the first and last part of the volume, I have written what I personally felt moved to write. These are my reflections, concerned to say what I needed to say at this particular moment in my life. I felt free to write thus in the conviction "that what is most personal is most universal", as Henri Nouwen puts it in the quotation on the frontispiece of this volume.

Perhaps it is necessary in this connection to say a specific word about the discussion of power in Chapter 9. Some readers may consider it extraneous, even inappropriate. I have lingered over that decision myself. But impending death does have a way of raising the question of power. How powerful, how dynamic has my life been? What forces for good have I helped to free in the world? In the end I decided that power issues, like funerals, are realities that need to be openly discussed.

Open discussion of power is, I think, especially needed in the ecumenical movement where the relentlessly waning power of the churches in the world has exacerbated the conflict in the ecumenical movement, a point elaborated in Appendix 3. I also hope that thus addressing the question of power openly may help to depersonalize the struggles in the ecumenical movement. It is, after all, against the "principalities and powers" (Ephesians 6) that we struggle, not against the persons ("flesh and blood") who are their often unwitting instruments.

Now as I write these introductory notes, I am at still another place. On my third trial run of chemotherapy, with the disease spreading rapidly, I know that this programme of treatment has about a five to ten per cent chance of being successful. I also know, partly because I have been able to write my way to it, that either way, if I live or if I die, my cancer has been overcome, as I hope my readers will perceive as they walk with me on this hard and cruel path.

I have not yet reached the end of that path. If this chemotherapy works and I live, then I might take a more systematic look at these experiences of the past few months. I would especially like to say something about doctor-patient relationships. In the course of such a chapter, I would need substantially to expand what I wrote earlier about my treatment. As I have written in Chapter 3, my in-patient care was outstanding. As an out-patient, however, I found the managing of appointments and the bureaucratic, procedural distancing of a highly specialized institution sometimes nearly intolerable. The medical care was still state of the art, but the focus seemed to be almost entirely on the *disease* rather than on the *person*.

I am indebted to many persons who helped these few testimonies into print: to Patricia Brouwer, Margaret Brouwer, Emalyn Reed, Onzalee Fanning, Gail Northrop and Nancy Alexander for manuscript typing and distribution; to Karin and Wesley Granberg-Michaelson for urging the WCC to publish; to Jan Kok for agreeing to do so and Marlin VanElderen for editorial assistance. Unnamed, but no less important, are all those who have supported me on the way and responded so graciously to these reflections in their original piecemeal form. I hope this publication as a whole will set these musings free to help others as they have helped me and those first readers.

Finally, a word about the appendixes. The "notes on ecumenical immobility" were put there to keep the main text clear of philosophical clutter (albeit *important* philosophical clutter). The sermons are closely related to the text of the reflections from which they spring and which at the same time they undergird and expand. Readers will notice that both sermons conclude with a quotation from Romans 8. Not all my sermons do! But it is one of the great New Testament statements of faith — and it is that faith which is the essential subject of these reflections.

July 14, 1993

Publisher's note:
On October 7, 1993, Arie Brouwer died. A funeral service
was held in Sioux Center, Iowa, on October 11; and there
were memorial services at the Ecumenical Centre in
Geneva and the Interchurch Center in New York, where
he had worked, and at the Community Church in Glen
Rock.

1. Discovering a Malignant Tumor

Pastoral care means offering your own life experience to your fellow travellers...

Henri Nouwen
Creative Ministry

December 20, 1992, 10:00 a.m.
The Fourth Sunday in Advent

For several days now I have been wanting to record some of the feelings, thoughts, reflections, insights that have come to me during the course of the past week. This hour of worship seems to be just the right moment.

First, a few facts for the record. Several days before my annual physical examination at the end of November, I began to feel a bit nauseous. There was also a heavy feeling behind my eyes. I attributed it to the flu then on the rampage, although I remember saying that I hadn't ever experienced anything like this except after eating tainted food or drinking impure water during my travels.

During the examination, my doctor felt what he thought was an enlarged liver and tested for hepatitis — negative. Ten days later I was back, still in pain. He sent me for an ultrasound test on the gall bladder — also negative. Next was a CAT scan of the liver on Wednesday, December 9. By that time I was beginning to feel ever-increasing pain. The CAT scan showed an enlarged intestine. A colonoscopy on Friday, December 11, revealed a malignant tumor, which was removed by Dr Ronald White on Sunday, December 13, the operation ending just about the time I had been expecting to begin the service at Glen Rock Community Church.

Dr White found a tumour about the size of a lemon pressing against the appendix, which was probably what caused the pain, thus alerting me to its presence. He removed both the appendix and the tumor, together with about 25 centimetres of colon and fifteen lymph nodes, six of which proved to be malignant. He also removed one of four spots found on the liver and performed a biopsy on another. Both of these proved to be malignant. These test results we received on Thursday night, December 17, shortly after I returned home from the hospital. They confirmed what I had expected.

The days in the hospital had provided opportunity to assess what I and my family were facing — in all likelihood a hard struggle against an enemy within. But what kind of struggle? This was not an enemy that could be outsmarted, outmanoeuvred, wrestled to the ground, overcome. This was an enemy that had to be "forced" out by what the eighteenth-century Scottish preacher Thomas Chalmers called, in his most famous sermon, "The Expulsive Power of a New Affection". This was an enemy to be "defeated" not only by medical means but also by the loving, healing power of God flowing into my life directly, without mediation, as well as through the loving, healing community of family and friends whose grace even in these days, perhaps most of all in these days, is sufficient for all my needs.

Cancer is of course a matter of the body as well as of the mind, the spirit, the soul, the emotions, so I wanted the best doctors — the pioneers — and the best possible environment in which to carry on the struggle. My doctor Jeffrey Lefkowitz understood that. "We will do everything medically and surgically possible for you," he said. "But finally it is your faith that will win this struggle." I told him then about my old friend Habakkuk, on whose message I had preached the second Sunday in Advent under the title, "Faith in Spite of Everything"!

At the moment therefore I am filled with gratitude — for the love and caring and strength and sheltering with which my wife Harriet and our youngest daughter Pat, who lives near us, surround me every day; for an excellent physician-surgeon team; for being next door to Sloan-Kettering Memorial Hospital where I will begin next week; for the tumor's obstruction of the appendix (a gift from God); for the gentle but persistent questioning from Pat and our son Milt, to make certain that Harriet and I know from the doctors all we need to know.

And I am grateful to be facing this struggle in the context of a pastoral ministry, whose nature is to deal with the issues of life and death and meaning and transcendence and where the things of God are transparent, rather than in the bureaucratic world, where even in the midst of the best of human relations it is not in the nature of things to discuss matters of ultimate personal meaning. They must rather be inserted by an act of will. I am grateful, too, for the particular people with whom I am ministering, the Community Church of Glen Rock. They have loved me to overflowing, supported and cared for me with a depth of feeling beyond my imagination.

No doubt they and other friends have noticed that these days I am often on, and beyond, the verge of tears. I have never been particularly uncomfortable about men crying, but then I've not made a public habit of it either. Why now? What does it mean? More things, I think, than I yet know. Before surgery, it was the pain. After surgery, it was again the pain, the shock to the system, the feeling of being invaded, not only by the surgeon's knife but by that strange secret enemy cancer — "the word most feared by Americans", one friend said.

Sometimes I have cried alone, but usually in the presence of people who love me, especially when one of them says something unexpectedly touching, and most of all in the presence of people who surprise me with their love.

For example, a member of the Glen Rock Community Church whom I had visited in the hospital twice in early December. He prayed for me all night, he said, and all through surgery. Just before surgery he called to give me a blessing: "The Lord bless you and keep you, Arie; the Lord make his face to shine upon you and be gracious unto you, Arie; the Lord lift up his countenance upon you and give you peace, Arie." A few days later he gave me what he called one of his most precious possessions, a small brass statue of the resurrected Christ modeled on the famous figure standing above the harbour in Rio de Janeiro. It sits on my bedstand now.

Or Dr Lefkowitz. Out of town at a seminar on the weekend of my surgery, he visited on Tuesday afternoon. I dutifully began exposing my incision, remarking that I supposed he wanted to examine it. "No", he said, "I came here to see *you*!" An act of love and caring made even more remarkable by the impersonal culture of this massive metropolitan environment in which we live.

Or Steve, my youngest son and father of my now almost nine-month-old granddaughter, saying, "Dad, twenty years from now I could have expected this, but I want you to be around for Rachel's graduation from college."

Or Charla, my oldest daughter, saying, "Dad, I've always felt a special relationship with you; and if you're not there, I won't have that special relationship with anybody." All these of course are strong incentives to love and to live.

I was astonished two days later when I learned that Charla was coming home (from Virginia) — and a little concerned whether I could handle it. I needn't have worried. It was a life-restoring visit, one more opportunity to love and be loved, to care deeply for one another with a clarity, I think, never before achieved.

All this is good. The crying, the cleansing, the loving, the healing — the power of love and the will to live and life itself all being exquisitely and inseparably inter-twined.

People fear cancer, and they find it hard to know what to say to someone who has it. Some say, "I'm sure you'll be all right." Or, "I'm sure everything will be all right." That bothered me. It seemed to drain the substance out of many of the other fine things these same people had said. How could they know? These words struck me as a kind of bland and blind optimism which was out of touch with reality — a view of life for which there is little if any room in the soul of this Dutch Reformed mystic. On the other hand, these were remarkable people making such state-ments. Fine people. Could they be right?

Gradually, it came to me that for some this may be just what it seemed at first to me: an empty optimism meant to keep life at a distance and despair at bay. But for others — sometimes knowingly, sometimes unknowingly — I think it is a profound statement of faith. Even if the tumor does prove to be malignant, even if you do have cancer and, yes, even if it is inoperable, untreatable and incurable, you will be all right, because you have lived your life by faith. Yours has been, is and will be a meaningful life, even a fulfilled life — a life filled full — while at the same time a life cut off and not completed. That is, I think, what even those who can do no more than deny despair are really trying to say.

So these have been rich days, full days, days of learning and acquiring wisdom. They have not been days of fear or depression or anger or anxiety. Neither Harriet nor I is afraid. We are not depressed. We are filled with hope and faith, yes, and even joy. We are surrounded by love — buoyed up on a gentle ocean of love.

"The waiting is the hardest," people have said to us again and again and again. Until now it hasn't been. When we were told the tumor was malignant, we were not surprised. We both expected the test results to be what they were. Now we both expect the liver to be operable, treatable, curable. We don't know. We may be wrong this time. We won't know until after Christmas. So as Advent draws to a close we are waiting, in the spirit of Habakkuk and in the spirit of the psalmist in whose words the Community Church of Glen Rock began its worship last Sunday, using the liturgy I had prepared but was unexpectedly unable to lead:

> We wait for the Lord,
> More than those who watch for the morning,
> More than those who watch for the morning.

2. Settling into the Struggle

December 27, 1992, 10:00 a.m.
First Sunday after Christmas

The life-threatening nature of cancer keeps pressing itself upon me these days. Mostly that stems from the cards and letters I am receiving in a wonderfully unending stream. They remind me that my illness is more than a matter of recovering from surgery, which is the way I myself am most aware of my body these days. In post-operative terms, I am doing very well. The pain is mostly gone, leaving in its wake enough discomfort to make recovery from surgery seem to be the thing that matters. As the signs and symptoms of bodily trauma fade, it seems that I am getting well.

The cards and letters remind me that I am *not*, that unrelated to the discomfort I feel there is another force at work within me, leaving no trace or feeling at all while it worries away at my life — at me. It's hard to believe — not to accept, to *believe*.

But it is there. The doctors are clear about that too. Last Wednesday was our first consultation at Memorial Sloan-Kettering Hospital. A sobering day from start to finish. The tumor, said Dr Turnbull, was a very aggressive one. There is no way of knowing how long it had been doing its work — perhaps five weeks, perhaps five years. No way of knowing either how far it has spread, but no doubt that it has. A scan of the lungs that afternoon would tell us more, as will a bone-scan next Wednesday. But for the liver itself, there is no way to know until surgery is in progress, at which time the surgeons will have to make some decisions about treatment, the options for which Dr Turnbull outlined.

Even if the affected part of the liver can be removed, the possibility of non-recurrence is only about 40 percent.

Absorbing that statistic, we didn't think to ask about the odds if a liver resection is not possible or about the survival rate for those in whom it does recur. (We did ask those questions by telephone a few days later. The odds for recovery grow less with each recurrence; they are also less if the liver proves to be inoperable.) Even with this later information we still have only statistics, not answers. If eventually the answer is healing, it will come only in God's good time. Meanwhile we wait for analyses and prognostications and statistics. The illness is elusive.

One of the decisions to be made in the next days is whether to take part in a clinical research project which involves placing a pump in the abdomen to feed the liver a slightly different chemical from what would be used in systemic chemotherapy. If they cannot operate on the liver, the pump is automatic; if they can operate, it is random. Does one choose the pump in the conviction that it may help, as it seems to have in the case of inoperable cancer? But if we choose it in hope, then what is the feeling if the random choice passes us by? (We decided to choose it.)

These are now the issues of our daily lives — our Christmas and New Year conversations — while the love flows back and forth between and among us each and all in a gracious warmth even richer than that we have known before. As I listen to my children's fears and concerns and anxieties, it dawns on me as well that it is in many ways harder for them than it is for me. True, mine is the life at issue, but it is my life to finish, if necessary, in the best way I can. For them, and for Harriet, it is a different question. If necessary, they too can each "finish" their relationship with me over the next weeks and months, but only in part — and then they will need to deal with an empty place. Even in this age of rampant individualism, there are still few words more bleak than "fatherless" and "widow". But we know these things. We are facing them. And we are finding strength and love, above all love — and laughter too.

Nor has any of us given up. Where love is, there is also the spirit of life. I want to live, to love and be loved, to celebrate life with wife and children and family and friends and neighbours. Sometimes in moments of pain or weariness, I have shrunk from the struggle, but only for a moment. I want to live.

Nor is either Harriet or I yet convinced that the Lord is through with me! I am still dreaming dreams — of a renewed church, of a better world, of an ecumenical movement made flesh in local parishes which would open themselves in faith to the whole height and breadth and depth of the entire Christian tradition, to know the presence of God as God cannot be known in any other way.

I have been made keenly aware of the abounding richness of that tradition again in these days as people have written and called to say they are praying for me. They number in the hundreds now, with many hundreds more drawn in through the prayer circles and congregations to which my family and friends belong. Through my friends at the World Council of Churches, these spirit-connections are linked across the continents until soon I suppose they will circle the globe.

Already they span the whole spectrum of the spirit — each with its own particular blessing. Take, for example, the prayers of the Orthodox and the Quakers. I suppose they are as different from one another in doctrine as it is possible to be while still naming the name of one Lord, holding to one faith and being united in one baptism. But they are bound together by being the church of the epiclesis (invocation), as the Orthodox are known, and the community of the inner light, as the Quakers understand themselves. With all their differences, they are closely akin in their awareness of the Spirit — and that is what matters in these things that matter the most.

Between these two points on the spectrum and even beyond them on either end in all the other communities of faith are many other friends who walk in the Spirit. Their prayers, too, I cherish as each appears before me uniquely in cards, letters and phone calls. This, for example, comes from one of my most beloved friends, not exactly orthodox, but full of the Spirit:

> So what do we say? We'd all like to fix this but of course we can't. So we each talk to our favourite spirits, powers or gods asking for help with your struggle and the return of physical health.
>
> The news came to me this morning, and my thoughts have been with you all day. Soon my friends will all know, and they'll be thinking of you too. And we'll send all the cosmic energy we can muster in your direction.

But I must take care not to suggest that intercessory prayer is somehow an esoteric activity fully available only to those who have cultivated a life in the spirit. No, here as in all other things, love is what matters. This is uniquely true for the Community Church at Glen Rock. If I were not now their pastor, I would still have been loved by many hundreds of people, but there would have been no community of love — at least not in that vital, even essential, physical sense that is now available in the Community Church. My other friends are scattered across the country and around the globe. These friends will be there Sunday after Sunday in the same place for me and for one another in the weeks to come. I can go home to them. It is an unparalleled gift of grace.

I remark it now again, because even though I continue to call these notes excerpts from my occasional journal, my friends know that my journals have been very occasional indeed. Can it be accidental that I again wanted to write while the service of worship was in progress at the Community Church? No, this is as truly the second letter to the church at Glen Rock as are any of the letters in the Christian scriptures to the churches loved by the pastors of that time. I marvel that this bonding of a few short weeks (I began my work there on October 1) could give me so much — and draw so much from me — but I do not doubt it to be true. And I am deeply grateful.

As I am for the community of clergy. At the hospital they stopped in one by one. As I told them my troubles, they nodded knowingly well before I had finished my story. They had been through it all before with members of their congregations, while I had been living out my vocation in the somewhat rarefied atmosphere of church bureaucracies — rarefied at least as far as this particular kind of personal human suffering is concerned. I drew strength from their wisdom. I gladly heard their prayers, so different from one another: some of them full of theology, others overflowing with personal caring, each blending these and other elements according to the gifts given to them, all of them means of grace. I am glad to be one of that company of pastors again.

My predecessor at Glen Rock, Vern Dethmers, is now in Florida and so knew only little of that we have passed through. But he summarized it well on the telephone yesterday when he said, "In spite of all that's happened, you are still in the right place at the right time." For me, that is certainly true. In a few weeks I'll be back preaching again, doing my best to make it true for the Community

Church as well as I bring them a gospel more fully mine to give away than ever it has been before.

January 4, 1993

Two good Mondays. Last week we got word that the lungs were clear; this week the bone scan came back clear. It is possible by faith to hope against hope, but it is easier when there are signs of hope.

3. Deciding about Surgery and Chemotherapy

January 12, 1993, 11:00 p.m.
Memorial Sloan-Kettering Hospital, New York City

Awakened by my nurse a little while ago for some medication before the surgery, I am now sitting on my bed waiting for it to do its work before I drop off to sleep again. Outside the night is foggy, filled with pinpoints of light: white, gold, blue, red — stationary for the most part, but some of them streaming both ways over the Williamsburg Bridge.

I think of Van Gogh's "Starry Night", which has long fascinated me, in part because in my near-sighted childhood before I wore spectacles that is how the starry night looked to me — huge globs of blurry light. Thinking of how often in the past few months I have been seeing the world through the eyes of artists and how rich an experience that is, I would like to paint this scene. "Foggy Night", I would call it, subtitled, "A Near-sighted Vision of the Williamsburg Bridge on a Foggy Night before Surgery". Well, maybe the sub-title should not be quite that long. But it would include a reference to the surgery. It clarifies, enhances, beautifies, nuances. I think again how much richer my life story will be because of all this, and I hope that the story will go on. Then I watch the night for a while, with and without my glasses, before once more in my mind saying "good night" to all those I love most in this life and drifting back into sleep.

January 13, 1993, 9:30 p.m.
Memorial Sloan-Kettering Hospital, New York City

How can news be hard and soft at the same time? This was the penultimate day we had been waiting for, intensely, the last couple of weeks: the result of the angiogram. We have it now. Multiple lesions in both lobes of the liver and inflamed lymph nodes. Sobering, altogether sobering. But we still don't know, as we knew we wouldn't, what is operable and what not. It is just that we had hoped the news today would reaffirm hope rather than pit hope against hope.

Dr Turnbull's primary concern now is the lymph nodes. If they prove to be malignant, then the operation will cease because the chemotherapy will need to be systemic. If not, then he may still be able to do a liver resection, depending on the size and location of the lesions. So again, it's tomorrow.

Happily, tonight I could talk with Milt and Steve in Ann Arbor, Michigan, and Char in Virginia Beach, Virginia, tell them this story and, as I had already done with Pat yesterday, reaffirm them each with the words I most wanted to leave with them before this operation. I cried it out then with Harriet and Pat. Somewhere amidst the tears my resolve was again renewed and I found the word I had been looking for: not to *fight* the cancer, but to *overcome* it. "'We Shall Overcome' is our song," I said. "We are not afraid." "We are not alone," said Harriet. The next weeks and months will no doubt require many an additional verse.

I know I shall need to draw on Harriet's indomitable spirit which seems never to waver. When confounded by the facts, she seems simply to change strategies. I wonder if she has ever retreated. In the face of this illness, I will have to learn from her how not to do that. From cancer there seems to be no such thing as a strategic retreat.

One of the hardest things will be to invest all that time in learning about cancer, the special diets, etc., etc. I say "invest," but it feels like "lose" — losing time and energy and vitality in chemotherapy. Somehow I need to discover the grace in this. Already in these reflections I see glimmers of that, but I am still a skeptic. I'll need to deal with that — but tomorrow, or a day or two after that. First I need to know the enemy's strength.

Meanwhile, I am drawing strength for myself from friends old and new, including Charles Young and Sue Berensen and Mercedes Condy (the last two friends of friends who have become friends) here at Memorial Sloan-Kettering and a wonderfully competent, patient and forthcoming staff who answer our questions without fail, while providing expert care with a remarkable quality of personal investment. What in most places is the exception seems here to be the rule.

January 24, 1993
Teaneck, New Jersey

No reflections for a few days. Well, actually lots of reflections, just no written ones. I came home from the hospital a week ago Saturday and before I had a chance to regroup was laid low by a post-operative intestinal infection. The pre- and post-surgical antibiotics killed off the good bacteria, leaving room for a very unfriendly variety to grow. I'm on my way out of that particular wood now — wanting to write and not wanting to write, so trying it out.

Curiously, the decision about chemotherapy has been the hardest of all. I thought I had made it before surgery, but that was a far less virulent, more specifically targeted kind. What is required now, without the liver resection, is a full-scale attack on my own body. Its redeeming feature is that it attacks hardest the fastest-growing cells, of which cancer is one type — and hair follicles another.

I had not known that that is the nature of chemotherapy. Now that I do, I don't like it very much. I hate it.
I have never taken anything on a regular basis, not even
vitamin tablets. I don't want to open my body to this awful
stuff. That is how I have been feeling these last few days.

With those feelings on the table, I wanted the feelings
on the other side to be just as open. What would happen if
I did not take the chemicals, if I relied on diet? What
would it feel like if that did not work?

Tuesday I started my day with the same resolution I
made on Monday: to learn all I could about chemotherapy.
But it didn't work. I couldn't seem to read or even to pick
up the book. So I let it not happen, and the other side of
my feelings began to play themselves out, all the way
through the hymns I would want sung at my funeral,
beginning with that soulful lament of Dutch Reformed
pietism, " 't Hijgend hert" (Psalm 42), entry music for the
life I now live and for my homegoing, concluding with the
triumphant shout of the Orthodox on Easter: "Christ is
risen!", "He is risen indeed!", entry music for the life that
is to be and for my homecoming.

And then I saw clearly, amidst the celebration, the
sadness, the emptiness, the loneliness, of those I love
most in this life that the celebration I most wanted was life
— with them.

My criteria are very simple. However short or long
the time I have, I want it to be the best possible quality,
for myself and especially for those I love most in this
life. I want to be present to myself and to them,
mentally, emotionally, spiritually, and as fully as possible. I want to finish working out the meaning of this
experience for my faith, to tell that good news to my
children and others who in their love for me cannot find
a workable answer to "Why?" As soon as I can handle

that emotionally in the pulpit, I want to preach that gospel. And if "closures" should become necessary sooner than they would in the natural course of life and death, then I want to be there, as fully as possible, as life passes through death into life.

Wednesday I met again with the chemotherapist, all 29 questions in hand and dealt with. As I listened, I began to think that chemotherapy might after all provide the best possible means for meeting my criteria. Thursday that still seemed to be the case, confirmed in a family conversation that night. So, I have decided to follow an experimental programme of chemotherapy that has produced good results (up to 70 percent) with other forms of cancer and is now being tested on colon cancer. If that fails, there is always the "conventional" treatment.

It is a curious thing that among the hardest issues to deal with is the so-called "side effect" of hair loss. It's only temporary and hardly lethal, but nevertheless extremely difficult emotionally. I suppose that is because it is the most obvious side-effect: the round-the-clock, undeniable, inescapable, flagrantly public announcement of my "condition", the most visible of all the attacks on one's personal dignity inherent in the treatment of this terrible disease.

But I am going to do it — a few weeks later than I thought because of the post-operative infection, which now makes me impatient. I want to get on with it.

Having decided, I want to relate my treatment with chemotherapy to what I believe. I want to accept this as a gift from God. Puzzling over that the other day, there suddenly leapt to mind last Sunday's "anointing" service. L'Anni Hill-Alto, pastor at the Pompton Reformed Church, had offered to conduct such a service in December. My immediate response was that I wanted it but thought that I would need it most after the second operation. So she came last Sunday with other clergy friends to sing and pray and listen and love and then to anoint with oil: my mind for clarity, my heart for courage, my hands for service, my wounds for healing. Can it be that Taxotere and 5FU and Leucovorin and all those other awful chemicals are also "oils" that are gifts from God? I'm not yet sure, but I'm working at it.

And I'm thinking... about the liturgies I'm going to create, about the sermons I'm going to preach, about the good news I'm going to give away when, in a few weeks, I return to the pulpit at Glen Rock. That in itself is a great gift, unique I think to pastoral ministry: to be able to work out the meaning of these experiences, not on the sidelines of life in ever more rare leisure moments, but as part of my common vocation with a community of believers who are working on similar and related questions.

4. Why?

We are often tempted to "explain" suffering in terms of "the will of God." Not only can this evoke anger and frustration, but also it is false. "God's will" is not a label that can be put on unhappy situations. God wants to bring joy not pain, peace not war, healing not suffering. Therefore, instead of declaring anything and everything to be the will of God, we must be willing to ask ourselves where in the midst of our pains and sufferings we can discern the loving presence of God.

Henri Nouwen
Show Me the Way

February 4, 1993
Teaneck, NJ

Driving back from a post-surgical check-up shortly after Christmas, my son Steve put this question: "When you were in the hospital, Dad, you talked about faith. What did you mean by that under these circumstances?"

"That even faced with this terrible disease, I live my life by believing in God, Steve. Why do you ask?"

"Because I can't figure out why God would let this happen. You and Mom too have devoted your whole lives to trying to make this a better world for people to live in. This is a strange way to be paid back. I know God doesn't *make* this happen. But why does God *let* this happen?"

"I have been thinking about that a lot too, Steve, and I've come to the conclusion that the old categories of God's 'prescriptive' will and God's 'permissive' will don't do the job. I am no longer satisfied to say that even though God doesn't cause my cancer, God allows it. I am persuaded that God does not want me to have cancer. I now think it happens anyway because God can't keep it from happening.

"I need to ponder that some more, but that's the way it seems to me now. I want to read the Bible again with that question in my mind. I want to dig into my theology books to examine again the basis for this idea of God's almightiness. But right now it seems to me that God can't keep this from happening."

"That's pretty much how I see it, too," said my son the theologian.

In the press of dealing with a second operation, post-surgical infections, learning about chemotherapy, diets and mind-body connections, I haven't done that digging yet. But I will, before my Lenten sermon on the fourth word from the cross, "My God, my God, why have you forsaken me?"

The "why" question came up last Friday night in David Frost's public television interview with Billy Graham. I wanted to watch the interview. I have rubbed elbows with Billy here and there around the country and around the world, and I like him a lot, even while disagreeing with much of what he says and does. Differences notwithstanding, I have found him more than once to be a channel of grace to me, personally.

It was a good interview, important enough to be written up at length by Peter Steinfels in yesterday's *New York Times*. The part that fascinated me was David Frost's pressing of the "why" question. "What would you say to the parent of a child with Down's syndrome? What about your own Parkinson's disease?" Billy gave the old answers: "God allows this to happen; he doesn't cause it to happen." He acknowledged though that he "didn't have all the answers" and that he had "a lot of questions to ask God when I see him face to face".

For most of my life I too had accepted, if not being fully content with, the mystery of God's will as encompassing all the events of our lives. And it had worked. I recall especially the time I was asked to speak with someone very close to me whose wife had been killed in a terrible traffic accident from which he had escaped virtually unscathed. He had stopped going to church. I soon found out why. "God needed her more than you did," his pastor had told this widowed father of one small child and a baby. Under the circumstances, telling him that God allowed it to happen only for reasons we don't understand was at least better news than he had heard before. He went back to church and a new life.

But now a decade and more later, that too seems like old news — or maybe no news. It surely is not good news. And it doesn't work for me any more, partly because it doesn't work for the people who love me.

Easing into the theological examination for that Lenten sermon, I decided to start with Howard Kushner's book *When Bad Things Happen to Good People*. I had known of the book, but I hadn't felt a pressing personal need to read it. Now I did. The surprises started on the dust-cover, where I read that Rabbi Kushner "learned that God is not the source of tragedy yet he hasn't the power to prevent it" — my own conclusion exactly. For him that insight was born out of parental anguish over the death of his fourteen-year-old son; mine was born out of personal illness. I devoured the book.

When I discussed this the other day with one of my dearest friends, she said, yes, she had read the book in the face of an earlier painful loss and it had helped her come to terms with God. It had also helped her to learn how to pray — what to pray for and what not to pray for.

It is a good book, I think, good enough for me to take the unprecedented action of ordering copies for each of our four children. It may help them to have these words coming from someone other than their father. It does seem to me that here and there, particularly in the chapters on pain and human freedom, Rabbi Kushner comes dangerously close to the old rationalizing ways. I think I will want to go a bit further than he, as well I might, following the way to which he himself points: "Christianity introduced the world to the idea of a God who suffers..." (p. 85).

On the other hand, Rabbi Kushner has already gone too far for some, like the friend I met the other day at a local delicatessen. No talk about the weather (coldest of the season). No small talk at all. "Arie!" she said, "I am thinking of you all the time these days, but not in this frame of reference!" Straight into meaning we went — cancer, prayer, Rabbi Kushner, God's almightiness or lack thereof. "I still haven't come to terms with my mother's death," she said. "But it's hard for someone brought up the way we were to accept Kushner's solution."

Yes, I'm sure it is. But I have found it liberating. I can be angry at my illness, at all the restrictions it is putting on my life, at the emotional cost it is extracting from me and Harriet and our four children, at all the extra freight it forces Harriet to carry. I can be very angry about that without being angry with God. In fact, I can trust that God is no less angry than I, perhaps more angry. What else is the meaning of God's wrath, but anger at sin and evil and suffering — to consume them and to leave in their place a world overflowing with justice and peace?

And what after all is sacrificed? It doesn't help much to believe in God's almightiness if the necessary corollary is that at the moments in life when that power of God is most needed, God may disappear into the vast remoteness of omniscience and omnipotence. My heavenly Father, revealed in Jesus Christ and present in the Spirit, does not withdraw. My heavenly Father identifies — most especially in my suffering.

March 19, 1993
Teaneck, NJ

I've done my biblical and theological spadework now. And this is what I have found (with the help of Theodore Jennings' wonderful book on the Apostles' Creed, *Loyalty to God*.) First, that God's almightiness is spoken of only ten times in the New Testament and that all but one of these references are in the book of Revelation. Looking at those texts, including the one in Corinthians, I found that every one has to do with God's ultimate triumph in history: that at the end of history God's love and justice and peace and well-being will prevail. And in the interim, God is with us in the struggle.

I said to myself then, "Arie, why in the world haven't you understood it that way before? This new understanding is entirely consistent with the whole teaching of the Bible that God created the world good, that sin came into the world and that the whole history of the world is God's struggle against sin in order to re-create for us the kind of world that God created for us in the first place. Why didn't you understand it that way in the beginning? Why hasn't the church understood it that way from the beginning?"

Perhaps it is because our creeds begin with the words, "I believe in God the Father Almighty...", leading us to think of God's almightiness in an abstract a priori sense, when these creeds are really statements about the work of God in history. And all of God's work in history is fulfilled only in the end time. The early centuries of the church, when these doctrines and creeds were being formulated, was a time of political absolutism; and in such a time perhaps one way to check the emperor's absolute power was to project a God even more absolute — and remote, high and lifted up, reigning supreme in the heavens. And perhaps it is because in those early centuries, Greek philosophy provided a concept for precisely such a God: the absolute abstraction of Aristotle's unmoved mover, an impassive God, unaffected by history.

With these old answers, as with Rabbi Kushner's new answers, we must raise the question of faithfulness to the biblical witness. The answer will soon be found. The idea of such an apathetic God will not survive even a casual reading of the scriptures. The Hebrew scriptures are no less clear than the Christian scriptures. God is a God of righteous deliverance, a God of the poor, a God of the exiled and the captive. God becomes angry with the people of Israel. God laments over the people of Israel. God's heart is broken over the people of Israel. The message from Genesis to Revelation is then not only good news for tomorrow, that God will ultimately triumph. It is also good news for today, that God is with us in our suffering.

Long ago Horace Bushnell asserted that a child growing up in the church should never know himself or herself to be "other than a child of God". That has been my experience. I recall it now in terms of some of the hymns I have especially treasured at various stages of my life: "Jesus Loves Me", "God of the Prophets", "God of Grace and God of Glory". From love through service to justice and hope. My whole life has been a love affair with God. I do not intend to give that up just because I have cancer.

5. The Relativity of Time and the Transfiguration of the World

February 4, 1993
Continental Flt. 479
Newark, New Jersey, to Phoenix, Arizona

I am on my way to visit my brother Lou and sister-in-law Esther in Arizona for a week of rest and recuperation in the sun — by the pool, I hope, weather permitting. Preparing for this trip yesterday and this morning, I recalled a conversation long ago with a colleague. We were sharing our experiences of how much work we were able to accomplish on airplanes and how it was often our most creative work — away from telephones and meetings and the other interruptions of the office. "But it's more than that," she said. "It's the altitude as well." She went on to claim that being physically raised above our usual environment somehow makes us able to transcend it and sets free our creativity. It was an insight new to me, but it rang true.

Now as I write, I am aware again that it is mostly at such special moments of transcendence that I want to write these reflections, whether today, lifted up by this Airbus 300, or on occasions when I know that the congregation I am now serving as interim pastor is gathered in the presence of God for Sunday morning worship.

Transcendence may also be nearly the right word for my new relationship with time. The subject came up again the other day in conversation with a clergy friend. He recalled what I had said during the anointing service a few days earlier about the new ways I am seeing beauty and joy and love and life itself in the people and the world around me. It is as if I have been given a kind of inner sight that sees the good things in our world, God's world, with a depth and breadth of vision not previously known. He reported that he had said to one of our mutual friends as they drove away from the anointing service that Sunday, "We should feel the same way. Our lives may be no longer, even shorter, than Arie's. We could wind up wrapped around a tree or in a head-on collision any moment."

"True," I said, "but it's not the shortness of time. I don't know either how long I have. It's related to time, but it's not time. It's something more I can't articulate just now. I need to think about it."

Now, as I write, it's coming clear. With cancer in my body, I know that the power of death is at work within me. I know it in a way I have never known it before. I know it with a heightened sense of awareness not even possible to imagine before. That awareness it seems is offset, perhaps transcended, by an openness to perceiving and receiving the gifts of life. Those gifts are everywhere — they always have been — but I now seem to see them against a contrasting background of death. The power of death within me does not dim the light of life; the power of death accentuates the light of life by sharpening the contrast.

All this is due not so much to time being short as it is to time being transcended. Time is not so much the agent that creates this change, as it is that which is acted upon by this different way of looking at life against the contrasting power of death. Against that background life is seen in the light of eternal life and time becomes relative. The relativity of time which I have begun to experience is setting me free from the seeming absoluteness of time. It is the awareness of that relativity which makes it possible to look ahead to what may be a short time without feeling despair. Even in a short time, life can be fulfilled.

Yesterday's mail brought a quotation from John Updike's *Self-consciousness*. It arrived in a letter from a friend, who had taken it from the letter of a friend, who in turn was quoting another friend who had also been stricken with cancer a few months ago. Such are the networks that spring up in the face of cancer! Updike seems to point in the same direction as my own musings: beyond the shortness of time to its relativity, towards a new way of perceiving time. The change is quantitative, to be sure, but mostly it is qualitative. He writes:

> I am now in my amazed, insistent appreciation of the physical world, of this planet with its scenery and weather [and] that pathetic discovery which the old make that every day and season has its beauty and its uses, that even a walk to the mailbox is a precious experience.
> I have the persistent sensation, in my life and art, that I am just beginning.

I know those feelings, including that feeling "in my life and art, that I am just beginning". There is something new about my life and my gospel these days.

Later in the day I discovered that it was not just one word I had been seeking but two. After having written the notes above, I had begun reading a book purchased last week at the Princeton University art museum, where Harriet and I had gone to see a display of Russian Orthodox icons, "Gates of Mystery". It was a magnificent exhibition, transporting the spirit. The book was Michel Quenot's *The Icon: Window on the Kingdom*. "The icon", he writes, "fulfills our vision of a universe of beauty by being a representation of transcendent reality." And "the icon... is the prototype... of our future transfigured humanity" (pp. 148, 150).

To the word "transcendent", then, must be added the word "transfigured". When you know first hand, in your own body, the encounter of death with life, the world is transfigured. The spiritual reality that constitutes the essence, the inner core, of every created being is more accessible than it has been before. You see things more nearly as they really are rather than as they merely appear to be. It is, I suppose, not unlike the gift given to the painter who can perceive and portray the inner being of a subject, a dimension the camera cannot quite reach except perhaps in the hands of an artist. But as Quenot says of the icon, this is not just a matter of art, but of theology (faith) and spiritual vision first of all.

The point is well made by Timothy Ware in *The Orthodox Church*:

> The world, as Gerard Manley Hopkins said, is charged with the grandeur of God; all creation is a gigantic Burning Bush, permeated but not consumed by the ineffable and wondrous fire of God's energies.

In "Aurora Leigh", Elizabeth Barrett Browning writes of both the inner and outer sight of which I have been speaking here:

> Earth's crammed with heaven,
> And every common bush afire with God,
> But only he who sees, takes off his shoes —
> The rest sit round and pluck blackberries...

I do not of course claim that I live in the fullness of that inner light all the time or even most of the time. I am only reporting that in the last few weeks it has illuminated my vision in ways that previously had been beyond the boundaries of my experience. And with John Updike, I am treasuring those moments of "amazed, insistent appreciation" of the world — already fleeting as I begin again to take up the tasks of daily life, of plucking blackberries.

Supplementing my reading still later in the day with Anthony Ugolnik's *The Illuminating Icon*, I found yet a third word that seemed to me to complete the circle:

time is transcended;
creation is transfigured;
relationships are transformed.

All relationships. From those with the persons closest to me all the way to the far reaches of my own experiences of the world. I belong to them, they to me, and all of us to God in a way not previously experienced.

I had taken Quenot and Ugolnik as my travelling companions because I wanted to keep alive the afterglow of that wonderful exhibition, "Gates of Mystery", at the Princeton art museum. I had hoped, too, that they might illuminate the sermon I will preach on my first Sunday back at the Community Church, which is Transfiguration Sunday. They will. I will of course deal with the gospel story of the transfiguration of Jesus. Then I will tell the congregation that during the past ten weeks I have seen them transfigured. I have seen more clearly than ever before the inner spiritual reality that constitutes the essence, the inner core, of this community of faith. They have demonstrated it in an outpouring of love and caring and spirituality beyond what I could possibly have imagined. I have seen it as well in the clergy, colleagues and friends who have come to support me personally as well as to carry on the ministry to and with this congregation.

Transfiguration, it seems, is also the right word to describe the expressions of love and appreciation from people whose lives I had touched long since in now mostly forgotten ways, only to discover in their letters during these days that many of those contacts had been full of meaning for them, meaning of which I had not been aware — or at least no longer remembered.

Perhaps most powerful of all are the letters from people whom I have known and loved for many years who, because of my encounter with cancer, have reached deep within themselves to understand and express the bonds that bind them to me and me to them. I want now to pursue those beginning explorations in long conversations which I know will further transform those relationships. I am certain, too, that in those conversations we will now and then glimpse the dawning of transcendent moments that will leave us transfigured one to the other — and light up the world around us.

6. The Funeral as Final Offering

May 15, 1993
Teaneck, NJ

During all the twenty-five years that I have been out of the pastoral ministry I have looked back on it with longing for some of its richer moments. Most precious in memory were the times for Bible study, reading and reflection, preaching and teaching. Richest of all, however, were the experiences of being with people at the moments of their deepest joy and most profound pain, especially births, weddings and funerals.

Nevertheless, when my thoughts have turned to funerals I have usually also remembered how uncomfortable I often was with the liturgy. No doubt the resurrection note with which it began was intended as an affirmation of faith amidst grief, but it was too abrupt. It left no space for public mourning. Further, the service was too short and, particularly when conducted in a funeral home, mostly without music (although the rubrics allowed that *"here a hymn may be sung"*).

In more or less that same grudging spirit of concession to American folkways, it was allowed that *"it may also be appropriate to acknowledge this hope as it was manifested in the life of the one who has died in the faith"*. To be sure, funeral eulogies too often render the persons eulogized unrecognizable to those who knew them, but in most lives there are at least some gifts of nature and of grace that may and indeed must be celebrated, not merely acknowledged. From such celebration, it seems, preachers tend to shrink, perhaps because they are afraid of being thought naive.

Even more fundamentally, the tradition itself seems to have shrunk from celebrating the lives of the departed, perhaps afraid that this might encourage a judgment on the deceased potentially more favourable than that to be pronounced by the Judge of all the earth! But that is not our affair. We are charged only, and are able only, to give thanks for those gifts and graces that have enriched our lives. We should do it with abandon and rejoicing.

Many times during my 25 years of work in the bureaucracy, these thoughts have wandered in and out around the edges of my mind. And many times I thought that I should develop the liturgy for my own funeral — as several of my friends had long since done. But I didn't. Partly because my funeral was not in my pending file, while many other things were; partly because I was never satisfied with the half-formed liturgies I did conceive only in my mind while on the run; partly, I suppose, because the life to be celebrated in my funeral was still in process of formation.

All these things I now see in a different light. During the last weeks, I have thought often of my funeral — and heard the music play. During the last few days I have given some hours to working out a liturgy for what it seems to me a funeral ought to be — and, specifically, for my own funeral.

Underlying and outweighing the dissatisfactions I have already mentioned — too abrupt a beginning, too short a time, too little music and too reluctant a commemoration of the departed — was the feeling that the funeral liturgy lacked a sense of movement. Yet a sense of movement is essential to any liturgy worthy of the name and most particularly to any liturgy that seeks to serve so fundamental a rite of passage as death and burial.

It is precisely such a sense of movement that I have striven to incorporate in the liturgy I have now developed. There are in fact six movements which I here sketch in outline and then discuss in detail.

ORDER OF WORSHIP FOR A FUNERAL SERVICE

We centre in the Spirit

Entrance music from the "Ikon of Light" by John Tavener
  Agios o Theos
  Mystic prayer to the Holy Spirit
  Agios o Theos
't Hijgend hert (two versions of Psalm 42 in Dutch)

The Lord's Prayer (in Dutch)

We mourn the passing of our brother Arie and lament our broken relationships

Pastor: Come to me, all you who are weary and are carrying heavy burdens, and I will give you rest. Take my yoke upon you, and learn from me; for I am gentle and humble in heart, and you will find rest for your souls (Matthew 11:28f).

People: Out of the depths I cry to you, O Lord!
          Lord hear my voice!
     Let your ears be attentive to my supplications!
          I wait for the Lord, my soul waits,
          and in your word I hope;
     My soul waits for the Lord
          more than those who watch for the morning,
          more than those who watch for the morning.
          (Psalm 130:1f,5f.)

Lamenting our broken relationships

A prayer for those who mourn

The hymn: "Seeking Water, Seeking Shelter"

We affirm the faith by which our brother Arie lived and witness to our own

Scripture readings: 2 Corinthians 4:1-2

> Therefore, since it is by God's mercy that we are engaged in this ministry, we do not lose heart. We have renounced the shameful things that one hides; we refuse

to practice cunning or to falsify God's word; but by the open statement of the truth we commend ourselves to the conscience of everyone in the sight of God.

Amos 5:24

But let justice roll down like waters,
and righteousness like an everflowing stream.

Psalm 27:1,3

The Lord is my light and my salvation;
whom shall I fear?
The Lord is the stronghold of my life;
of whom shall I be afraid?
Though an army encamp against me,
my heart shall not fear;
though war rise up against me,
yet I will be confident.

Romans 8:37-39

No, in all these things we are more than conquerors through him who loved us. For I am convinced that neither death, nor life, nor angels, nor rulers, nor things present, nor things to come, nor powers, nor height, nor depth, nor anything else in all creation, will be able to separate us from the love of God in Christ Jesus our Lord.

Hebrews 11:32-38; 12:1-2

And what more should I say? For time would fail me to tell of Gideon, Barak, Samson, Jephthah, of David and Samuel and the prophets — who through faith conquered kingdoms, administered justice, obtained promises, shut the mouths of lions, quenched raging fire, escaped the edge of the sword, won strength out of weakness, became mighty in war, put foreign armies to flight. Women received their dead by resurrection. Others were tortured, refusing to accept release, in order to obtain a better resurrection. Others suffered mocking and flogging, and even chains and imprisonment. They were stoned to

death, they were sawn in two, they were killed by
the sword; they went about in skins of sheep and
goats, destitute, persecuted, tormented — of whom
the world was not worthy. They wandered in deserts
and mountains, and in caves and holes in the
ground.

Therefore, since we are surrounded by so great a
cloud of witnesses, let us also lay aside every weight and
the sin that clings so closely, and let us run with perseverance the race that is set before us, looking to Jesus the
pioneer and perfecter of our faith, who for the sake of the
joy that was set before him endured the cross, disregard-
ing its shame, and has taken his seat at the right hand of
the throne of God.

John 14:1-7,18-19,25-27; 16:12-13
"Do not let your hearts be troubled. Believe in God,
believe also in me. In my Father's house there are many
dwelling places. If it were not so, would I have told you
that I go to prepare a place for you? And if I go and
prepare a place for you, I will come again and will take
you to myself, so that where I am, there you may be also.
And you know the way to the place where I am going."
Thomas said to him, "Lord, we do not know where you
are going. How can we know the way?" Jesus said to
him, "I am the way, and the truth, and the life. No one
comes to the Father except through me. If you know me,
you will know my Father also. From now on you do
know him and have seen him."

"I will not leave you orphaned; I am coming to you.
In a little while the world will no longer see me, but you
will see me; because I live, you also will live."

"I have said these things to you while I am still with
you. But the Advocate, the Holy Spirit, whom the Father
will send in my name, will teach you everything, and
remind you of all that I have said to you. Peace I leave

36

with you; my peace I give to you. I do not give to you as the world gives. Do not let your hearts be troubled, and do not let them be afraid."

"I still have many things to say to you, but you cannot bear them now. When the Spirit of truth comes, he will guide you into all the truth; for he will not speak on his own, but will speak whatever he hears, and he will declare to you the things that are to come."

Psalm 27:4
One thing I asked of the Lord,
that will I seek after:
to live in the house of the Lord
all the days of my life,
to behold the beauty of the Lord,
and to inquire in his temple.

Witnessing to the faith (concluding with the Apostles' Creed)
The hymn: "God of the Prophets"

We celebrate the life of our brother Arie and give thanks for the gifts he gave us
Scripture reading: Ephesians 4:7,11-16

But each of us was given grace according to the measure of Christ's gift.

The gifts he gave were that some would be apostles, some prophets, some evangelists, some pastors and teachers, to equip the saints for the work of ministry, for building up the body of Christ, until all of us come to the unity of the faith and of the knowledge of the Son of God, to maturity, to the measure of the full stature of Christ. We must no longer be children, tossed to and fro and blown about by every wind of doctrine, by people's trickery, by their craftiness in deceitful scheming. But speaking the truth in love, we must grow up in every way into him who is the head, into Christ, from whom the whole body, joined and knit together by every ligament with which it is equipped, as each part is working properly, promotes the body's growth in building itself up in love.

Giving thanks for Arie's gifts to us

The hymn: "God of Grace, God of Glory"

We envision the homecoming of our brother Arie as he joins the great parade

Scripture readings: Psalm 84:1-4

> How lovely is your dwelling place,
> > O Lord of hosts!
> My soul longs, indeed it faints
> > for the courts of the Lord;
> my heart and my flesh sing for joy
> > to the living God.
> Even the sparrow finds a home,
> > and the swallow a nest for herself,
> > where she may lay her young,
> at your altars, O Lord of hosts,
> > my King and my God.
> Happy are those who live in your house,
> > ever singing your praise.

Revelation 7:9-17; 21:22-26

> After this I looked, and there was a great multitude that no one could count, from every nation, from all tribes and peoples and languages, standing before the throne and before the Lamb, robed in white, with palm branches in their hands. They cried out in a loud voice, saying,
> > "Salvation belongs to our God
> > > who is seated on the throne,
> > > and to the Lamb!"
> And all the angels stood around the throne and around the elders and the four living creatures, and they fell on their faces before the throne and worshipped God, singing,

"Amen! Blessing and glory and wisdom
and thanksgiving and honor
and power and might
be to our God forever and ever!
   Amen."

Then one of the elders addressed me, saying, "Who
are these, robed in white, and where have they come
from?" I said to him, "Sir, you are the one that knows."
Then he said to me, "These are they who have come out
of the great ordeal; they have washed their robes and
made them white in the blood of the Lamb.

For this reason they are before
      the throne of God,
   and worship him day and night
      within his temple,
   and the one who is seated
      on the throne will shelter them.
They will hunger no more,
      and thirst no more;
   the sun will not strike them,
      nor any scorching heat;
for the Lamb at the center of the throne
      will be their shepherd,
   and he will guide them to springs
      of the water of life,
and God will wipe away every tear
      from their eyes."

I saw no temple in the city, for its temple is the
Lord God the Almighty and the Lamb. And the city
has no need of sun or moon to shine on it, for the
glory of God is its light, and its lamp is the Lamb.
The nations will walk by its light, and the kings of the
earth will bring their glory into it. Its gates will never
be shut by day — and there will be no night there.
People will bring into it the glory and the honor of the
nations.

Envisioning Arie's homecoming

The hymn: "For All the Saints", stanzas 1,2,4,5,6

The benediction

More entrance music: *Funeral Ikos*, John Tavener

We commit the body of our brother Arie to the earth and its Creator

Scripture reading: 1 Corinthians 15:35-58

But someone will ask, "How are the dead raised? With what kind of body do they come?" Fool! What you sow does not come to life unless it dies. And as for what you sow, you do not sow the body that is to be, but a bare seed, perhaps of wheat or of some other grain. But God gives it a body as he has chosen, and to each kind of seed its own body. Not all flesh is alike, but there is one flesh for human beings, another for animals, another for birds, and another for fish. There are both heavenly bodies and earthly bodies, but the glory of the heavenly is one thing, and that of the earthly is another. There is one glory of the sun, and another glory of the moon, and another glory of the stars; indeed, star differs from star in glory.

So it is with the resurrection of the dead. What is sown is perishable, what is raised is imperishable. It is sown in dishonor, it is raised in glory. It is sown in weakness, it is raised in power. It is sown a physical body, it is raised a spiritual body. If there is a physical body, there is also a spiritual body. Thus it is written, "The first man, Adam, became a living being"; the last Adam became a life-giving spirit. But it is not the spiritual that is first, but the physical, and then the spiritual. The first man was from the earth, a man of dust; the second man is from heaven. As was the man of dust, so are those who are of the dust; and as is the man of heaven, so are those who are of heaven. Just as we have borne the image of the man of dust, we will also bear the image of the man of heaven.

What I am saying, brothers and sisters, is this: flesh and blood cannot inherit the kingdom of God, nor does the perishable inherit the imperishable. Listen, I will tell you a mystery! We will not all die, but we will all be changed, in a moment, in the twinkling of an eye, at the last trumpet. For the trumpet will sound, and the dead will be raised imperishable, and we will be changed. For this perishable body must put on imperishability, and this mortal body must put on immortality. When this perishable body puts on imperishability, and this mortal body puts on immortality, then the saying that is written will be fulfilled:

"Death has been swallowed up in victory."
"Where, O death, is your victory?
Where, O death, is your sting?"

The sting of death is sin, and the power of sin is the law. But thanks be to God, who gives us the victory through our Lord Jesus Christ.

Therefore, my beloved, be steadfast, immovable, always excelling in the work of the Lord, because you know that in the Lord your labor is not in vain.

Committing Arie's body to the earth

(As the body is committed to the grave, earth may be cast upon the coffin by the minister and/or the family and friends of the deceased.)

Into your hands, O merciful Saviour, we commend your servant, our brother Arie, and now commit his body to the (earth from which it was made/ deep/ elements/ this resting place), earth to earth, ashes to ashes, dust to dust, in sure and certain hope of the resurrection to eternal life through our Lord Jesus Christ, at whose coming again in glorious majesty to judge the world, the earth and the sea shall give up their dead; and the corruptible bodies of those who sleep in him shall be changed, and made like unto his glorious body;

A prayer for those who are bereaved

Let us pray.

Eternal God, Creator and Giver of life, in the beginning you formed us from the dust of the earth and breathed into us the breath of life. So also, you have promised in the end time to raise us from the dust, to which we must return so that we may assume a new body at the coming of your Son. Make us strong now in this hope which you have kindled within our hearts, that our brother Arie, who has died, will be raised to life imperishable.

Father of mercies and God of all comfort, we pray that now in this present moment of grief you will look in your tender love and pity, on all these your sorrowing servants. Enable them to find in you their refuge and strength, a very present help in trouble; help them to know the love of Christ which passes knowledge. Grant them faith and hope in him who by death has conquered death, and by rising again has opened the gates of eternal life, even Jesus Christ our Lord.

Ever blessed God, we give you thanks for all the generations of the faithful, who, having served you here in godliness and love, are now with you in glory. We praise you especially for him whom you have now taken to yourself, this pilgrim now come to the heavenly city. For all your loving kindness towards him throughout his earthly life we give you thanks. For all that he was, by nature and by grace, to those who loved him and to the church of your dear Son, we praise your name. We thank you that, his trials and temptations being ended, sickness and death being passed, he has now entered into the rest that remains for your people.

Seeing that we are surrounded by so great a cloud of witnesses, enable us, O God, to lay aside every weight, and sin which clings so closely, and to run with perseverance the race that is set before us, looking to Jesus, the pioneer and perfecter of our faith. Keep us in unbroken fellowship with the church in heaven; enrich our souls in

those things over which darkness and death no longer
have any dominion; and bring us at last, with all the
faithful in Christ, to the eternal peace and joy of your
presence; through Jesus Christ our Lord; in whose name
we are bold to say:

The Lord's prayer

The hymn: "How Blest Are They Who Trust in Christ"

The Apostles' Creed

The benediction

Now may the God of Peace who brought again from
the dead our Lord Jesus, the great Shepherd of the sheep,
by the blood of the eternal covenant, equip you with
everything good that you may do God's will, working in
you that which is pleasing in God's sight, through Jesus
Christ; to whom be glory forever and ever. And the
blessing of our Triune God, Father, Son and Holy Spirit
be and abide with you always. Amen.

The first movement of this liturgy and any other is that
of centring in the Spirit. The Spirit, I believe, is present in
the tradition, which, as the great Orthodox theologian
Georges Florovsky always insisted, is a charismatic principle rather than merely an historical record.

For my own service I have drawn first from the music
of John Tavener, which I have only recently discovered.
However new to me, I have used it here because Tavener
draws on the music of the Orthodox liturgy to render
profoundly moving and exquisitely beautiful modern music
— thus representing the charismatic principle of renewing
the tradition by following the Spirit. I have chosen it as well
to symbolize my own deep indebtedness to the Orthodox,
particularly since 1980. Tavener's music appears again at
the end of the service as "More entrance music" — this time
to the next life — because its ethereal heavenliness seems to

me the best bridge available to the world we do not yet know. Having decided on Tavener, I discovered these two pieces almost by accident, purchasing the compact disk without any knowledge of its content. I cannot now imagine a more sublimely beautiful expression of longing for the Holy Spirit — so important to me — or a more exquisite statement of open-eyed realism about death, combined with deep faith about the future, and at the same time recognizing fully that while we believe much, we know nothing about the world that is to be.

The heart of this first and centring movement is, however, from my own tradition — from the psalm most treasured by the Dutch Reformed pietism I inherited from my father and particularly from my mother. I often sang the 42nd psalm with her while my brother struck its long notes on the family piano. I treasure it all the more because the only recordings we have of my parents' voices are of them singing psalm 42 and praying the Lord's prayer.

To my mind the passionate spirituality of this psalm in Dutch surpasses even that of the Hebrew and is not at all evident in the English version sung at the end of the next movement in this service. The difference I think will be obvious to anyone comparing the following translation of the first verse of the Dutch psalm with either the hymn "Seeking Water, Seeking Shelter" or the text in the Bible itself. The passion of the Dutch version I claim as my own.

> As the panting hart
> pines for the clear water,
> my soul cries out to find God,
> whom I look for breathlessly.
> Yes, I seek his countenance,
> God of life, God of light.
> When shall I praise him again,
> and stand jubilantly in his courts?

The second movement is for public mourning. It begins with a loving invitation from our Lord, opening the way for a cry from the depths. The public mourning that follows is articulated either by the pastor or by a friend of the family who knows the nature, number, variety and pain of the broken relationships.

The third movement affirms the faith incarnate in the life of the departed. Here I have woven together some threads of Scripture to which I have often clung for support. Psalm 27:4 stands apart and at the end because I have just now discovered that its statement of life's "one thing... to behold the beauty of the Lord and to inquire in his temple" sums up exquisitely the nature of my pilgrimage, which centres in an ever-growing love for beauty (greatly stimulated by the Orthodox, for whom beauty is a theological statement) and an ever-probing quest for truth as the fulfilment of faith. I would want these passages to be read by someone skilled in inter-pretative reading and then supplemented by the words of two or three friends with whom I have witnessed side by side.

The hymn "God of the Prophets" was written in 1884 by a minister in the Reformed Church in America for the centenary of New Brunswick Theological Seminary. It appears here partly for that reason, but mostly because it best expresses the spirit of this particular facet of my life — which has been the guiding principle in the selection of all the music.

The fourth movement is a celebration of, by and for the people. Following the Scriptures, which are again interpreted by being read well, a few persons chosen in advance will lead the thanksgiving, after which the pastor will invite a brief word from anyone else who wishes.

The fifth movement consists again of Scripture and a brief statement from the presiding pastor reflecting conversations we have had during these weeks concerning the life to come, thus bearing witness to our Christian hope in the resurrection.

The sixth movement takes place at the graveside and consists of readings from Scripture and the liturgy, a hymn and a second recitation of the Apostles' Creed, which is never more clearly a statement of faith than when spoken beside an open grave.

* * *

For some time I felt a certain ambivalence about whether this plan for a funeral service belonged among the entries from my journal selected for publication. Then I read Carl and Stephanie Simonton's book *Getting Well Again* (which I return to at length in chapter 10). They describe an "imagery process" in which their patients took part, intended to give them new perspectives on life and death. Among the reactions of the patients were "imagining their funeral" and "formulating an idea of how they wanted their funeral to be conducted". Reading that convinced me that I should include this chapter. Death is an inescapable part of our human condition. That underscores once again Henri Nouwen's reflection on the self-portraits painted by Rembrandt, which I have chosen as the epigraph for this book: "Rembrandt realized that what is most personal is most universal."

7. Forms of Support

June 3, 1993
Teaneck, NJ

My family members tell me that I am handling this illness with courage and independence. I keep feeling as if I need mountains of support. In any event I am getting it — from many, many people.

First and foremost among these "caregivers" is Harriet. I don't know how she does it. She has held her present full-time job for less than a year, so she is still learning the systems at her office while at the same time installing new ones. Caring for our day-to-day living requirements at home is another full-time job — with no help at all from me now. And there is yet another full-time job caring for me: listening, holding hands, hugging, supporting — trying to figure out what food to serve now that I have to eat more than ever just to sustain my weight, even though I often do not want to eat at all; sorting out all the medical bills and shepherding them through her insurance company; watching me struggle with pain and weariness while feeling totally helpless to do anything to change that; answering dozens of phone calls enquiring about my and her well-being. I don't know how she does it.

Most important to me is the listening, talking, holding hands, hugging and sometimes actually holding me while I cry out the pain and weariness and depression at the end of a hard day. We have talked about everything during these last weeks. I have sorted out and reviewed with her our financial records. We have rewritten our wills and then revised them again, changed property titles to avoid unnecessary entanglements with probate courts and judges and had some preliminary conversations about burial places, while at the same time struggling every day to keep hope alive for a continuing life together. I didn't think we could love each other more than we did, but we do.

My children, too, have been there for me, each in his or her own way: writing letters, telephoning, visiting (and while visiting helping out with the chores I can't do), taking me to consultations with doctors and to chemotherapy appointments, holding me amidst my tears, loving me.

Very close to that inner family circle are two nieces with whom I have had especially close relationships over the years for reasons we have glanced at but never explored. They are doing that exploration now in wonderful, deeply moving and sustaining letters. Soon we will continue those explorations in long conversations as they also come to visit.

One of them writes that for her I represent the "elder" in her family, "who most clearly shares my own values, hopes and dreams". I wept as I read that, remembering my own Uncle John, my father's younger brother, who broke the family mold of midwestern farmers and made a very different life for himself in California. I remember the excitement of his rare visits to us and my own visit to him with my parents when I was about eleven or twelve. I think then that I know what she means, what she feels and I glow with satisfaction.

The other niece writes that to her I "really feel like a second father". Again I draw a parallel from my own experience. I have been fortunate to have several such surrogate fathers who have enriched my life beyond telling. They have mostly been mentors whose most *obvious* gifts to me were professional, but whose most *precious* gifts were far more personal. Once again my spirit warms within me, and I am deeply grateful for these two young women, their love for me and mine for them and the mutual enrichment of our lives.

Just beyond my immediate family is the larger circle of brothers and sisters, in blood and in law. Next are the other nephews and nieces and their offspring — numbering well over 200, perhaps 300. Many of them have written, some several times. Particularly satisfying has been the continuing care of my five brothers and one sister and Harriet's four brothers and three sisters. We have lived a thousand or more miles away from them for most of the last forty years. Even though still separated by those distances, they have been in close touch during these past months, many times.

In the still larger circle of friends, it is the letter writers who take pride of place. Good, long, old-fashioned letters gracing my struggles with special treasures of love and appreciation. Sometimes these letters have moved me to tears, or brightened my life with satisfaction, or filled me with awe at the depth and quality of caring of those who have written.

Many of the letters have recalled and affirmed ways in which I have enriched the life of the writer. That's always good to hear, of course, but in the midst of a life-threatening illness in which I feel myself day-by-day face-to-face with death, it is doubly good — even more than doubly good. Some of these friends have shared an especially treasured poem, hymn, prayer or some other word or picture in the hope that it would mean as much to me as it does to them.

In response to my reflections there has come from time to time a loving nudge to keep a full-orbed perspective:

> Rest well, my friend. Prepare for the battles and struggles that are ahead of you. Be fully informed and totally realistic, as I know you are. But also from time to time, dare to hope for a miracle.

Many a letter has begun with a confession that the writer hardly knows what to say, or can't say what he or she feels, or doesn't know whether the letter will be mailed, having tried many times before to write. But they have written and they have posted the letters — and they have blessed me in doing so.

The friend quoted just above put it this way at the end of her two-page letter:

> I don't know what has made me go on at length — I don't know where you are in your treatments, and whether long letters are wearying. I guess it just seems that illness is a time for recounting the ties.

Yes, it is. Indeed, during the past few months I have often said to myself and to Harriet, even amidst my misery, that the hope one hears expressed so often that "when I go, I want to go quickly" isn't all it's reputed to be. In the midst of terminal suffering, yes, surely; but before that the time to "recount the ties" and to get a fresh grip on them before they are transformed is a rare and precious gift.

This gift has been given not only to me, but to my family as well. When they come to visit, they invariably ask, "Dad, where are the letters that have come since I was last home?" They want to read them, to know my life and my friends and what connects us and to savour it with me.

If, contrary to what I usually feel these days, death should come sooner rather than later, then those circles of love will help us all to face it. And if I live, they will provide an environment in which to pass along with stronger hands the values I have tried to live by. Either way, the letters are a priceless gift.

I suppose more than a few who have wanted to write have been frightened off by the feeling that they could not write what they wanted to communicate. Let me say that also among my treasures are simple greeting cards with a brief note of love or humour or whatever else. One person simply wrote, "I am not good with words, so we'll just let you know you are in our hearts and prayers." Another sent only a piece of notepaper that read:

> Dear brother Arie:
> I have been wanting to write you since the middle of December when I first heard of your illness.
> But I don't know what to say!
> Love and Peace

It, too, was enough.

I have particularly valued those simple greeting cards which have kept coming, week after week, month after month, from the same people — not with dramatically new words of wit or wisdom but with an abiding sense of unflagging caring and commitment. Such cards, letters and phone calls have continued to pour in by the hundreds every day now without a break for the entire six months of these struggles. That is many more than I expected. It is due, I think, to a number of unusual if not unique factors. I have already mentioned my exceptionally large family circle numbering in the hundreds. In addition, I have held highly visible positions in several large organizations. Further, in the months before this catastrophe, I had the good fortune to become interim pastor of a wonderful congregation.

Without such support, the struggle would be much harder. I have often thought that without Harriet's love I would have given up. Perhaps, perhaps not; there is no way to know. But I do know that I am deeply grateful to her and every other person who has taken time to care.

Having been an ordained minister for over thirty years, I naturally have a large circle of friends among the clergy. But, although most of these are pastors, none of them was *my* pastor. I wanted and needed one, someone who was not first my friend and then also my pastor, but someone who was first my pastor and who could then become my friend as well, someone with whom Harriet and I could discuss *all* the problems we were dealing with in total confidence and without any reservations about what that might mean for past or future relationships. I particularly wanted someone who could and would be there for Harriet in that uniquely pastoral role in the event that the cancer does win and takes me from her.

For that I turned to Lynn Van Ek, whom I had engaged as pastoral associate for congregational care for the Community Church shortly before I became ill. Unknown to me except through her references, she has proved to be a blessed gift to the congregation and to Harriet and me. She has helped us to identify our needs and equipped us with resources to meet those needs with unusual skill and empathy — never, for example, assuming that she knows our prayer needs, but asking us on every visit what those needs are before she offers her parting prayer.

The mention of resources calls to mind that the offering of resources is not always received as support. It can be a negative factor as well as a positive one. Because cancer is such an elusive disease, with no certain cures, there are hundreds, perhaps thousands, of possible or supposed "cures" in circulation. More than a few of them have found their way into my mail box. At first I found that very confusing and frustrating. In the face of cancer, I wanted to do all I could to defeat it. But I couldn't try everything.

Chemotherapy, strengthening my body's immune system, cultivating mind-body relationships, perhaps following special diets — these seemed to be the main approaches. Early on I decided to rely chiefly on chemotherapy combined with faith, while doing what I could with diet and perhaps trying a few folk cures along the way as bodily strength permitted (which so far it has not). I am content with that now, knowing that I am doing the best I can even while filing the information I continue to receive for future reference and for discussion with my doctors if present strategies fail and my strength makes possible yet another effort. In a few weeks, after yet another CAT scan, we'll know more; and if the present treatment is also failing then I think I will be glad to know that there is still something else to try.

8. Unfinished Business — Personal Relationships

June 10, 1993
Teaneck, NJ

For my Sunday sermon texts during Lent I used our Lord's seven words from the cross. I remember reading another preacher's sermon on the third word from the cross, "Mother, behold your son". The preacher went on at some length to express amazement that there, on the cross, Jesus should be thinking about his mother. He supposed only someone divine could think of another person under such circumstances.

I didn't think it amazing in the least, since it closely paralleled my own experience prior to surgery. I am well aware that surgery is no crucifixion. But I was in pain more severe than any in my life, and I knew by then that I was dealing with cancer in a potentially terminal form. Yet — or perhaps better *therefore* — my thoughts were all of Harriet. From the moment I heard the diagnosis on Friday night, a malignant tumor, to going under the anaesthesia, my thoughts were all of Harriet, and specifically of whether I had done enough to provide for her if she needed to finish out her life alone.

I had thought about that before, of course, but never as systematically and carefully as I should have and as I had done with most things in my life. There are many reasons for that. First, Harriet and I were married in the middle of the 1950s, when it seemed that the world (at least in the United States) was getting better and better. My own parents had come from deep poverty, struggled through the depression and finally made it to a comfortable old age, retiring from their farm in the early 1950s when my father was only 57, my age now. It seemed that we were virtually assured of satisfying work and a good life. Why worry about the future?

And then of course I was a minister, freed by my congregation — as the language of the letter of call put it — "from all worldly avocations". Further, I just couldn't get interested in money. I paid attention to it only when there wasn't enough to go around. As for the future, life had gone very well for me, far exceeding anything I had ever imagined in terms of satisfying, rewarding and exciting work, world travel, a globe-encompassing circle of friends and a wonderful family. Whenever we had been in financial straits we had always found a way out. When I thought about it at all, I found it easiest to think of my own skills and reputation as our security.

How radically all that had changed! First, my reputation had been badly damaged by the public attacks on me prior to my departure from the National Council of Churches. Now I was face to face with death. As it turned out, I learned in the weeks after surgery that with the life insurance benefits payable in the event of my death Harriet would be fine — a fact that comforted me greatly, even though it didn't mean much to her. She was reassured, of course, but she wanted only one thing — for me to live.

In these weeks after surgery, particularly after the second operation, which had struck a hard blow against hope (Chapter 3), we asked ourselves whether there was unfinished business between us: misunderstandings, uncertainties, whatever. We, mostly I, found a few things to clarify, in order to be certain that resolutions of old problems from years ago were still in place, that there was no guilt, that what had been resolved was truly resolved. They had been, and that was that.

Unfinished business with other people was not that easy. First, the children. We have always talked things through together, not only between Harriet and me, but with our children as well. Yet families are very complex institutions, in which we are at our most vulnerable, so that we seem unavoidably to hurt, wound or damage those we love the most — often by trying to help them! As our children grew, we had discovered some of these hurts and talked them through. But such conversations are not something done once for all. Lives keep unfolding. As the years pass, we discover more of ourselves and others, particularly of our parents; and in light of such new awareness we sometimes need to revisit former days. I had expected that to continue for at least another twenty years as my children grew into middle age and I into old age. Now it seemed that this might not be. Somehow we had to find a way to reach backwards and forwards at the same time, beyond our present levels of self-awareness, in order to do our unfinished business ahead of schedule.

We have done quite well, I think. We have found that the way to connect those dim pasts and unknown futures which we have not yet discovered is to probe as deeply within ourselves as we possibly can. Each of us has had to do this probing first on our own and then together as we sought the courage to speak of things of which we were only vaguely aware and therefore not yet truly ready to speak. That has been made much easier by our children's wonderful faithfulness in visiting, coming in from Michigan and Virginia to all be together at Christmas, in mid-February, again at Easter, yet again at the end of May for Memorial Day — and then in September on Labor Day to celebrate our 38th wedding anniversary.

Included in those visits have been the two newest members of our family: Margaret, Steven's wife of five years, and their one-year-old daughter Rachel Marie, our first daughter-in-law and first grandchild — two very special people. With Margaret it has been a very rewarding challenge as we have each discovered new dimensions of love in what is a new relationship for both of us. But however well begun, this is a task still mostly unfinished.

As for little Rachel Marie, the role of grandfather is one I especially cherish. I dream of reinventing and retelling the stories I used to fabricate for our own children, to be present with her parents at the rites of passage in her life, to explore what it means to be a grandfather. That strong anticipation of my own is much strengthened by her parents' strong desire for me to be there for their daughter. The unfinished dimension of this task I cannot even begin to imagine.

As I write these lines, I realize that all these matters of unfinished business are incentives to live, to overcome the cancer, to beat it back, to eradicate it from my body. I think, too, that this "obligation" to Rachel Marie, small as she is, has about it a particular joy that lifts my spirit, that moves me in a very special way to celebrate her life and, through her, all life.

Beyond that immediate family circle are the larger circles of family, friends and acquaintances. I was startled last week when I reread a January letter from a friend who wrote of Henri Nouwen's "need to set things right with everybody with whom he was angry when he thought he was going to die after being struck by the side view mirror of a van on a stormy day in Toronto". Since rereading that letter I have been asking myself whether there are people like that for me whom I need to see. There are a few, but they are people with whom I have often tried to work out our difficulties to no avail. I know, too, that there are people angry with me for one thing or another, but with each of them I have also tried, often repeatedly, to be reconciled, and again to no avail. They know the offer is still on the table, and these days I simply don't have the strength to reach out yet another time.

Over the past months, some of the people who have unfinished business with me have written to put matters right. A few have written to confess a wrong done to me, or to wonder if I am angry with them for what I may have considered a wrong done to me even though they hadn't intended it to be such. Sometimes I have had to struggle to recall what those wrongs might have been, and one or two I have been able to recall only with Harriet's help. To all, forgiveness asked has been freely given and recognized as mutual. In those cases where I am clear about the wrong done to me, such mutual forgiveness has been mostly a matter of assuring the other that for me the matter has long since been resolved. Nevertheless, this certifying of resolution, of forgiveness, is extremely important. Without it, the matter between us could not be truly and fully finished, wrapped up, thrust behind us both. It has been good of these friends to write.

Among the most touching letters have been several from people whose employment I have had unhappily to terminate in one or another position I have held. Not one of them has even mentioned that hard fact. Instead they have chosen to remember the good times, to recall how I have helped them or the satisfaction they had in working with me. It takes a lot of character to do that. Once again, it has been very good of these friends to write.

No matter how open, free and gracious these personal relationships become, they are of course never really finished. That would be true no matter how long one might live. Yet this is no cause for disappointment. Even after my death, whenever it comes, my family and friends will be able to go on "finishing" their relationships with me as a part of what the hymn-writer called "the mystic sweet communion with those whose rest is won". What I mean by that — and my own experiences of it — are dealt with at length in the sermon for All Saints Day which appears in this volume, so there is no need to spell it out here. I mention it only to finish this reflection on the general unfinishedness of life with a note of hope. No, more than a note, a *theme* of hope, an important theme that enables us Christians to see beyond the years to confess our faith in a life that transcends this one, of which such communion is one manifestation.

9. Unfinished Business — My Ecumenical Vocation

June 11, 1993
Teaneck, NJ

The daily flow of mail which has meant so much to me has brought a few troubling letters. Not many: fewer than a half dozen of the thousand-plus cards and letters. Curiously, all of them came from middle-aged or senior white men with whom my primary relationship was through the National Council of Churches. That may only reflect the fact that my time at the council was by any standard the most traumatic of my work experiences. I resigned in 1989, less than halfway through my second term as general secretary. But I suspect it also points to the guilty self-knowledge of "liberal" white middle-class males in the US that they tend to skirt issues rather than deal with them — a quality of character which I am afraid most ecumenical organizations provide abundant opportunity to cultivate. In any event, guilt is the unifying theme among these letters.

I want to reflect here on a subject raised in one of these letters, in which the writer intermingled a critique of my pursuit and use of power, as he saw it, with reflections on his own use, non-use and misuse of power, comparing his own impending loss of power as he faces retirement with the powerlessness I feel with cancer in my body. The exercise of power has been an important part of my life; and it is something on which I have often reflected in a variety of situations, though I have found few friends in the clergy who are willing to discuss this issue (a dangerous attitude, given the fact that ministers exercise power all the time).

I have often experienced the exercise of power as creative, redeeming and life-giving. One of the first things that sprang to mind when I read the severely negative judgments in this letter on the exercise of power was what may have been my own most assertive use of power: when I insisted that the ordination of several women in the Reformed Church in America be dealt with by the general synod in 1979 in a certain specific judicial framework. I believed then and continue to believe that the approach which I as general secretary helped to shape, advocate and implement was correct. I also believe that without my intervention, others would have sought again to diffuse the conflict by forcing it back into a legislative frame of reference; and the ordination of women would again have been defeated, as it had been for the previous thirty years. Had I not exercised such power, I would not have been able to receive the splendid pastoral care that has come to me from L'Anni Hill-Alto (the anointing service described in Chapter 3) and Lynn Van Ek (Chapter 7). How can I then think about that use of power as "petty and useless" — in the words of my correspondent.

My chief regret with respect to power is that I was not able always to empower the institutions I served so that they might in turn effectively serve their members and the well-being of the human community. Most notably, this was true of the National Council of Churches, where I had hoped to build on the regional offices of Church World Service an ecumenical network for peace, justice and the well-being of creation which would have given those offices more integrity while at the same time enabling the Council to be an effective instrument for the cultural, social, political and economic renewal of our disintegrating society. That is a major piece of unfinished business — with not the slightest prospect of completion in sight. One can only hope and pray that somewhere there are church leaders now in formation who will have the will, wit and wisdom to answer the call for the redemption of the world before it is too late.

I had also wanted to empower the churches by persuading them to create truly ecumenical programmes, which would be developed and administered together, rather than continuing to develop denominational programmes which were only sometimes cooperative and at best loosely coordinated. In their separateness, these programmes went largely unnoticed both in the power centres of the world and among the poor and oppressed whom they were designed to serve. It seemed to me that if these programmes were united, the world might take notice and the poor and oppressed might be blessed, as in the civil rights struggle of the 1960s which was an ecumenical effort.

This empowerment was also unattainable largely because the denominational programmes had become essential to the survival of the denominational structures. Only a few persons recognized that programmes designed to serve the structures were ultimately destined to atrophy and die — and the structures with them. Unfortunately, not enough of these persons had sufficient influence in their own denominations to take the risk of genuine ecumenical programme development, which might have breathed new life into the programmes and opened up a new future for the denominations.

Writing here of my unfinished ecumenical agenda naturally leads me to think of the World Council of Churches as well. The WCC was and is the chief instrument of my own ecumenical formation. That formation began in the late 1960s with my in-depth exposure to the WCC study on the "Missionary Structure of the Congregation". Throughout most of the 1970s I watched the WCC from afar, listening and learning. In January 1979 I succeeded to the WCC Central Committee seat of Marion de Velder, my predecessor as general secretary of the Reformed Church in America.

Central Committee membership was a key step in a fascinating and formative journey that led to my appointment in 1984 as a deputy general secretary of the WCC. That was a position I did not seek and did not want, but both Harriet and I felt that my ecumenical vocation required a yes. It turned out to be an exceedingly rich even if unusually brief relationship. Rich because of the wonderful people on the staff. Short because I became embroiled in the election of the next general secretary of the WCC by becoming a candidate for that position.

The Russian Orthodox were the first to raise the possibility of my serving as WCC general secretary. They did so indirectly with a US church leader friend who mentioned it to me well before I joined the staff. I considered myself qualified in terms of ecumenical vision and commitment as well as institutional leadership skills. At the same time, I thought myself to be so lacking in experience and familiarity with the leaders of the worldwide ecumenical community as to disqualify me. Moreover, coming from the US is often a liability in the international arena, the more so in this instance since one of the three previous WCC general secretaries — Eugene Carson Blake — had been from the United States.

After I joined the staff, the pressure grew; and I eventually agreed to be a candidate, a decision made with a mixture of reluctance and anxiety on the one hand and excitement and vocational commitment on the other. One of the two or three decisive factors in my decision was that I understood myself to be the preferred candidate of both the Russian and US representatives serving on the nominating committee. Only very late in the process —

during the last few hours of the nominating committee's work — did I learn that the Russians had long since changed their mind (but had neglected to tell me). If I had known of their decision, I would immediately have withdrawn as a candidate. I shared with some US church leader friends my disappointment with the Russians and together we decided to talk with them. We had no thought of changing the decision of the nominating committee but we did want to encourage more honesty and openness in international ecumenical relationships, a point I think the Russians were not able to accommodate because of their own complex and difficult relationships with the Soviet state.

A few months later when I was elected general secretary of the National Council of Churches, the Russians were more than a little anxious about the possible effect of this earlier misunderstanding on their relationship to the NCC. The NCC was their main link with the churches in the US and thus an important element in undergirding their status in the eyes of their own government, since their relationship with it opened a channel of communication to the West, particularly the US which the Soviet government sought often to exploit as a vehicle for its propaganda.

These anxieties were of course reported to me indirectly, through intermediaries; and I answered through the same channels, "not to worry". It was unthinkable to me that the church in the Soviet Union should be deprived of support and perhaps its members made to suffer in order to "punish" a few of their leaders.

The central public figure in the relationships of the Russian Orthodox Church with the WCC and the NCC was Metropolitan Philaret of Minsk, who chaired the Department of External Relations (the ecumenical office of the church). Already in the early 1980s I had made his acquaintance when I chaired the NCC's committee on US-USSR church relations. After 1985, when I served as general secretary of the NCC, I came to know him quite well. But in all our meetings, the painful confrontation at the WCC in the summer of 1984 was never once mentioned. Nor were any of our other confrontations over the policies of the US and Soviet governments. We preferred to toast our successes.

The confrontations about our governments' policies were of relatively low intensity, with one notable exception: the Moscow Peace Conference in May 1982. I remember those intense confrontations very well. They began in private meetings with Metropolitan Philaret before the conference began. I stressed that given the high visibility of this conference in the major US media, we could not afford to tolerate a propaganda blitz conducted by the Russian Orthodox Church or by churches in other Soviet-bloc countries in order to curry favor with the Soviet government. As always, we remained committed to speak the truth as we saw it in the joint communiques which we were accustomed to issuing at the end of our meetings. Moreover, since the media were likely to cover the day-to-day proceedings of the conference, we would need to insist on truth-telling throughout. I alerted Metropolitan Philaret and his associates that we would not shrink from openly challenging the conference while it was in progress, even to the point of publicly withdrawing if we came to feel that continued participation would endanger our credibility as peacemakers in the United States. That responsibility we could sacrifice, even for the well-being of the Russian Orthodox Church, since our primary vocation was in the US.

Some of those conversations were intense. But they were necessary. Indeed, on the very first day of the conference, it seemed clear to me and to other senior members of the US delegation whom I consulted that a public confrontation would be required. A steady stream of presentations was lopsidedly blaming the US and excusing the Soviet Union for the global problems related to the arms race.

Unknown to me, that was also the opinion of Bishop David Preuss of the American Lutheran Church. As a member of the presidium, he was invited to chair a part of the proceedings, and he registered those concerns as he took the chair shortly before I began my address to the conference on behalf of the US churches. Overnight I had inserted into my speech a call for a course correction; and since the text of the speech had been distributed in advance, the insertion was very pointed indeed. Although David and I had acted independently, our names were linked in media accounts which probably gave us more credit than we deserved for saving the conference.

There were serious reservations within the US delegation as to whether David and I had gone too far and thus endangered our relationships with the Russian Orthodox Church and their place in their society. I was therefore more than a little pleased to receive a letter from David in February 1993 in which he recounted a recent conversation with Metropolitan Philaret:

> We talked of the Moscow Peace Conference, and he told how he and other Russian Orthodox leaders looked at it as the great watershed in their relationship with the state. They had screwed up their courage and told the state authorities that they must keep out of the Peace Conference and let the religious people say what they felt they needed to say. He said the meetings with the US delegation had been crucial in

helping them face the state. He especially cited you as leader of the US delegation. From that time on, Philaret said, the church had space to live and work that it had not had for fifty years.

He wanted me to be sure to greet you, wish you well and assure you that you would be in his prayers.

Even though there is much ecumenical business left unfinished, something of great importance was accomplished. At this stage in my life, that is very satisfying to know — not just to believe, but to *know*.

It is good as well to know that truth-telling works, at least sometimes, even in this mendacious world where words have lost so much of their meaning. It is no accident that my last report to the governing board of the NCC was entitled "Stand for Truth". It was my ultimate challenge to us as a national council to face the truth about ourselves as we were always urging others to do — indeed as we were at that very time doing in relation to the government of South Africa, under that very same slogan: "Stand for Truth". Half of the board wanted to stand for the truth as I saw it and presented it. The other half did not. I decided it was pointless to continue the struggle, that I had done all I could, that the institution could not be "overcome" from within, so I resigned.

Writing about these items of unfinished ecumenical business reminds me that Lesslie Newbigin entitled his autobiography *Unfinished Agenda*. It reminds me as well that my friend Konrad Raiser, the new general secretary of the WCC, is calling for a new ecumenical vision. That is indisputably an urgent call, to which I hope the churches will respond. But I do not think they will, for several simple but powerful reasons (which I will elaborate in Appendix 3).

There is, I believe, one last best hope for the ecumenical movement, at least in the United States. That is the creation and cultivation of ecumenical congregations. The membership of most "mainline" congregations in the US already includes persons from many denominational backgrounds. For the most part, however, those potential ecumenical riches are not realized in the lives of the congregations. Unless the present process of diversification is given serious attention, we will be subjected to a kind of ecumenism by erosion, from which the distinctive elements of the various traditions have been leached. That will be a great loss, since most of those traditions have at one time or another in history served to fill in an inadequacy or correct an error in the dominant religious group. I dread to think of the bland and formless religious liberalism with which we will be left — and how it will be ravaged by the religious right.

But this phenomenon of plurality within more and more congregations offers an interesting ecumenical opportunity if the diverse traditions could be consciously articulated in congregational life (not just at the national levels of the denomination). If the particular contribution of each tradition to the fullness of the gospel (the Tradition) were acknowledged, affirmed and then integrated in a recognizable way into the life and especially the worship of the congregation, then I believe we would create congregations with a sturdiness and attractiveness that would give them a burst of new life, perhaps even ending the mainline malaise.

In short, I am suggesting that the way forward in the ecumenical movement is to be found in a movement from below. This has long since been true of the Christian base communities in Latin America. Rather than trying to duplicate these base communities in very different societies in the North, we must instead create the forms for such a movement from below that are appropriate to our own culture. In the US, I believe, that way forward is to be found in ecumenical congregations.

I have done a bit of experimentation with that possibility in the past few months while serving as interim pastor of the Glen Rock Community Church. Unfortunately, my cancer cut short the experiment; but in the first stages there was nothing but enthusiasm. From such ecumenical congregations could eventually grow a national Christian council that would gradually transform the anachronistic and divisive denominational structures that are now stifling the ecumenical movement. Deprived of their determinative divisiveness, the denominations could serve a function in such a council much like that of the orders within the Roman Catholic Church.

This is, of course, a dream, even a distant dream. But in it I find one more powerful incentive to live in order to experiment with it for the glory of God. Yes, for the glory of God. At bottom that is the essence of the ecumenical movement. However important for the movement are the unity of the church and the pursuit of peace and justice and environmental wholeness — and they are very important to the movement and to me personally — my ultimate commitment to ecumenism springs from the fullness of the presence of God which I have known within this movement as nowhere else. I have known this in community experiences of all kinds but most especially in worship. I long for all God's people to have that experience, and I would like to do what I can to enable it.

That longing is tied closely to one other: to re-articulate my faith — not in an academic theological work but in song and sermon and liturgy — in precisely such an ecumenical congregation.

There is much that is unfinished. But for me that is an invitation not to despair or somehow to cling desperately to life. Once again I have been helped in this by preaching my way through our Lord's seven words from the cross, particularly the penultimate word, "It is finished". What a claim! Preachers have often extolled it as unique to Christ's divinity. But then I remembered that Jesus too had more than a little unfinished business. Why, I wonder, did Jesus in an earlier word from the cross pass responsibility for his mother to a cousin, not to a brother. There are many possible reasons, but perhaps there were unresolved tensions in family relationships springing from that unusual scene in which he rejects his biological family, claiming his followers as his family (Mark 3:31-35; Matthew 12:46-50; Luke 8:19-21). Less speculatively, we know from John's record that Jesus had many things left to teach his disciples which they could not hear before his death (John 14:24f.; 16:12f.).

So what does it mean for Jesus to say, "It is finished". It means, I think, that Jesus had persevered to the end in his mission of truth and love. To the end, at the risk and cost of his life, he had told the truth about God, about the church and about the world. Not everything was finished, only his mission of love and truth.

I have tried to do that too. Even in this reflection on my own unfinished agenda, I have tried to speak the truth in love and hope about the ecumenical movement. And therefore, by the grace of God and in the face of all that is undone and all my mistakes and shortcomings and failures, and all I would like still to do, I also make bold to say, even with a loud voice, "It is finished", and then, quietly and at peace, "Into your hands, Father, I commit my spirit".

10. Healing and Faith

In general, people are quicker to believe in the relationship between dying and a negative expectancy than in the relationship between getting well and a positive expectancy.

Carl and Stephanie Simonton
Getting Well Again

June 28, 1993
Teaneck, NJ

The relationship between faith and healing is a subject I've been thinking about for years in a variety of contexts. How does faith heal? Is cancer a stress-related disease? My general assumption was that faith can and does heal. But why then does faith heal some and not others? Is it because the faith of some is too small, too weak? But doesn't that make faith itself a work? And doesn't that nullify the central tenet of Protestant Christianity that we are saved by faith and not by works?

These are a few of the thickets through which I have never made time to find my way. Now they are existential questions. The relationship of faith and healing, like the question of "Why?", has been on my mind almost non-stop since I learned that I have cancer. It was brought out in the open almost immediately by the statement of my doctor, Jeffrey Lefkowitz, "We will do everything medically and surgically possible for you, but finally it is your faith that will win this struggle."

Even before that, it was the subject of a sermon, "Faith in Spite of Everything", based on Habakkuk 3:17-19, one of the most beautiful lyric statements of faith anywhere in religious literature. I had written the sermon especially with a member of the congregation who had cancer in mind; by the time I preached it, I was convinced that I too had cancer, even though my doctors had not yet confirmed that. As it turned out, that proclamation of the message of Habakkuk was to be the first of several cancer-related sermons I was to preach over the next months.

Over those months, I have read a few articles and essays as well as Bernie Seigel's *Love, Medicine and Miracles* and *Peace, Love and Healing*. I've had more than a few conversations as well. But not until last week did I tackle the question systematically. On the top of my stack of books to read on the subject was O. Carl Simonton's *Getting Well Again*, written in collaboration with Stephanie Matthews-Simonton and James L. Creighton. It turned out to be a wonderful book, precisely what I needed to find my way through the thickets.

What I most appreciated about the book is its unflagging and rigorous commitment to honesty about cancer, the patient, the doctor, the family and other support groups. Also it deals directly with the question of guilt in the contexts in which it is most likely to arise, which I needed, because Seigel's books had increased the pressure on me to feel guilty if my faith didn't "work" and I didn't become one of the "miracles" and sometimes even made me feel guilty for giving myself cancer. The problem with Seigel's books, I think, centres in his making the cures "miraculous". He then makes the exception the norm (in his preface to the 1990 edition of *Love, Medicine and Miracles*, he calls his exceptional patients "normal") and seems to keep saying over and over, "*Believe, Believe, Believe*". Seigel tells the stories of his exceptional patients to reinforce these expectations. The Simontons, on the other hand, explore their patients' stories to see what can be learned about the body-mind connection.

Reading Seigel reminded me of the "self-help" best-sellers of the 1950s, which encouraged us all to think or believe our problems away. The self-help books seemed to encourage denial of the real-life physical and temporal existence of our problems. That worked for a lot of people, but not for me; my critical threshold is too high, my Calvinist realism too much on guard against pseudo-idealism.

The Simontons relate faith and healing by exploring the connection between faith and the body's immune system. They also take care to relate the cure of the disease to its causes in mind, body, spirit, emotions and the environment. Again and again, I found the Simontons articulating precisely and thereby brightening what for me had been only glimmers of truth as I tried to grope towards an understanding of the body-mind connection.

Reading the Simontons has set me free now to write my own thoughts and feelings about faith and healing and about body-mind healing. I have held off doing so because I have wanted to have something more to say than, "Well, yes, I think there is some kind of connection, but I'm not sure what it is." Often in these months, mulling these questions over, I have recalled the words of the man who responded to Jesus' statement that "all things can be done for the one who believes" with the cry: "I believe; help my unbelief!" (Mark 9:14-29). I think that for the first time, I understand that desperate cry.

Intuitively, I knew that the truth of which I had seen some glimmerings was larger than my questioning perception of it. But I couldn't reach it, picture it, articulate it. Now I know it empirically, factually, scientifically — not as a foundation for faith, but as a clarification of how faith works. What I see now fits well with my understanding of how God works in the world, not against God's own creation, but with it, to bring it to fruition.

Most if not all writers on mind-body healing emphasize the need to review one's life before the advent of cancer to discover particularly disturbing psychological situations which caused feelings of helplessness and hopelessness. Because almost everybody seems to know this, some of my friends have, I know, speculated about the degree to which my troubles at the National Council of Churches caused my cancer. I have wondered about that, too, because cancer has often seemed to me a stress-related illness. The Simonton book enables me now to say with certainty that those troubles did not *cause* my cancer, but they more than likely contributed to it. They argue that stress of the kind I experienced at the NCC weakens the immune system so that it is unable to fight the cancerous cells that are searching for places in our bodies most of the time. Thus, such an experience "does not cause cancer, rather it permits cancer to develop... by interfering with the immune system". Earlier, in Chapter 4, I explicitly rejected applying this dichotomy of "cause" and "permit" to an all-powerful God. But I am more than willing to accept this as a description of our finite immune systems, which "permit" cancer only because they are unable to prevent it.

I need to emphasize that I am not making this connection in order to create guilt in those who opposed me at the NCC or even those who attacked me personally. Opposition almost always clarifies the issues; personal attacks are matters to be dealt with quite apart from my cancer. Furthermore, I could have walked away from the NCC much earlier, or settled for an ineffective existence there. I chose to stay — for reasons I will discuss later — even though I knew it was very bad for me and often said to family and friends, "I need to get out of here before this job kills me." Moreover, there was more to my life than the NCC. So who is to say what "caused" what? Who is to say what "permitted" what? All I wish to state unequivocally is that I accept that these factors contributed to my illness; and I make this statement only because the factors that "permitted" or "caused" my cancer need to be addressed in curing or overcoming it.

The mind-body connection needs as much attention as the other factors that contribute to cancer. The real issue, say the Simontons, "is no longer whether the mind and emotions affect the course of treatment; the question is how to direct them most effectively in support of it." For me the central element in the mind-body connection is my faith. This is particularly true as faith bears on my "will to live", which in turn is central to mind-body healing. Simply put, the question is: Do I dare to hope?

To my own amazement, I have found that feelings of helplessness and hopelessness (which are closely related) can so permeate me and those close to me that we find it hard to believe good news when we get it! My last CAT-scan, for example, showed that my current programme of chemotherapy had arrested my cancer. We might on that basis have begun to believe that it has been stopped. But our questions sometimes overshadow belief. We have found that belief is easier for other people with whom we have shared that good news than it is for Harriet and me. On the surface that seems surprising. I do after all read body signs that point to the tumours continuing dormancy, even perhaps to its retreat. But there are other signs as well, and the bad news is easier to believe.

Taking a long look doesn't help either. Will I ever feel truly well again? If so, will I be able to find the work I want, a congregation in which to fulfill my ecumenical vocation? I have been among the most fortunate of people in having had thirty years of extraordinarily meaningful and significant work. Can I find that again? Or will I have to settle for something that will pay the bills? Is there any employer out there who will be willing to settle for a cancer patient? Will there be any work at all?

In the face of such questions, faith is the only durable foundation for hope I can find. Faith that God is a loving God. Faith that God is not only with me in my struggle for healing — and perhaps able to cure my cancer — but also that God will be with me in meeting the demands of living. Responding to critics who suggest that they may be offering people "false hope", the Simontons readily agree that there can be no guarantees; then they add: "Hope, we feel, is an appropriate stance to take toward uncertainty." Faith, knowing that God is with me, helps me to take that stance towards uncertainty and to maintain it in spite of the bad times.

Faith in a loving God also helps me to forgive myself for whatever I may have done to "permit" cancer to develop within me. I mentioned earlier the other options I had for dealing with the troubles at the NCC: walking away or settling for ineffectiveness. Those were options, but they were very difficult options, given my sense of vocation, my long association with and commitment to the NCC and my strong feeling that if the NCC once again backed away from its problems, it would not have many more chances to face them before it was so weakened as to be virtually meaningless. Hard options. They left me feeling trapped, not knowing how to find a way out for me or for the NCC.

Yet looking back now, I feel forgiveness for whatever errors and mistakes I made that may have contributed to this illness. For me, faith in a loving God makes such forgiveness possible. If God doesn't hold it against me, why should I? That is the real point of the fifth petition of the Lord's Prayer, which I think might well be translated, "Forgive us our trespasses *so that we can forgive* those who trespass against us." It is God's forgiveness of us that makes it possible for us to forgive ourselves and others. I believe that since I have done the best I could, my heavenly Father is satisfied. I feel forgiven, and for my healing that is what matters. Truth, after all, is larger than the mind. Essentially truth exists in right relationships, ultimately in right relationships with God. Such faith, such truth involves one in a continuing quest, beholding the beauty of the Lord and enquiring in God's temple, to recall the words of Psalm 27 used in my funeral service.

In a section entitled "Changing Your Beliefs", the Simontons say that

> our experience has shown that patients who have slowly, sometimes even grudgingly, altered their beliefs have done particularly well in our programme. The time taken in consideration and internal argument has allowed them to integrate their new beliefs into all aspects of their personality and behaviour.

So, theological reflection, theological struggle, theological wrestling, is important. It is another one of many instances where I have found that the course I have been following is precisely the one the Simontons prescribe.

To complete this reflection on the role of my faith and mind-body healing, I must include at least a note about the other factors that contribute to cancer. The Simontons are clear that their approach is part of a "whole-person model" of cancer recovery. Like Michael Lerner of Commonweal, a California-based centre for mind-body healing, they warn strongly against seeing mind-body healing as a substitute for standard medical treatment, insisting that the two be used together. The causes of cancer must be addressed, not merely the disposition that permits cancer.

The Simontons identify in particular carcinogenic sub-
stances, genetic predisposition, radiation and diet. Harriet
and I have attended to all those over the years except
genetic predisposition. I knew that my father had cancer
of the prostate before he died, full of years, at 83. The
same cancer was discovered in one of my brothers
recently, but contained. But I had forgotten that two of my
father's brothers had died of cancer. Fuller awareness of
these facts might have led me to opt for a colonoscopy in
my annual physicals, but maybe not, and we don't know
how long the tumour was there. In any event it is too late
to change that now; as Kierkegaard said, "life is lived
forwards, but understood backwards."

Knowing what I now know and being who I am, my
commitment — though sometimes admittedly a wavering
one — is to overcome cancer. Rereading the earlier
entries in this journal the other day, I discovered that in
my first entry I had rejected the word "overcome", along
with a string of other fighting words. In the third entry,
written only four weeks later, I had embraced it as the
right word to describe this struggle. It still seems to be
the right word, again reinforced by the Simontons' use of
it in the subtitle of their book: "A Step-by-Step Self-Help
Guide to Overcoming Cancer for Patients and Their
Families".

The word is, of course, familiar from that great
spiritual song of the civil rights movement, "We Shall
Overcome", and is thus indelibly associated in my mind
with Martin Luther King, Jr. Thinking about that the other
day, I was struck that King's focus was not on the enemy,
not on the dogs, the bullwhips, the firehoses, the white
hoods, or on those who used these instruments of oppres-
sion. His focus was on what lay beyond the struggle, on
"the beloved community".

Now as I write I recall suddenly that in the old King
James Version of the Bible the Book of Revelation is
sprinkled with the word "overcome" from start to finish.
Pulling down my concordance to check out my memory, I
discovered that it is the translation of the Greek word
nikao, which means "to gain the victory". Yes, of course.
The struggle is not to defeat the cancer; it is to gain the
victory, to inherit life in all its fullness.

The frequent occurrence of "overcome" in the Book of
Revelation had been almost expunged from my memory
because the Revised Standard Version translated it by
"conquer". Whether or not that is a more accurate render-
ing of the Greek, I am reminded just now, as I often am,
of one of the great transcendent passages of the New
Testament, the conclusion of the eighth chapter of
Romans, in which Paul says:

> No, in all these we are more than conquerors to him that
> loved us. So I am persuaded, that neither death, nor life, nor
> angels, nor principalities, nor powers, nor things present,
> nor things to come, nor height, nor depth, nor anything else
> in all creation, shall be able to separate us from the love of
> God in Christ Jesus our Lord.

That is the meaning of "overcome", not merely to lay
waste the enemy, but to enter into a wholly new relationship of well-being. In the language of body-mind healing,
to overcome is to be "weller than well", in other words, to
have discovered a range of life meaning that is much
broader, wider and deeper than we had known before.
That is what makes it possible to overcome even if one is
not cured and cancer becomes the instrument of one's
death. That is what makes it possible to claim the victory
even if death appears to be the winner, and to do so
without seeming to escape into pious mumble-jumble.

I do not know what shape death will take for me. I do not know what will be the final shape of my overcoming. I only know that already through the love of God in Christ Jesus our Lord, I am more than a conqueror. This is true even though I hardly know the outlines of the struggle. I do not know what form the enemy will take. The enemy is elusive. (Even in the midst of writing this particular reflection I had to be rushed to the hospital for tests to see whether I had a pulmonary embolism or merely pneumonia or bronchitis. It was diagnosed as the latter.)

But I am ready now, as the Simontons suggest, to create my future, to set some goals. Perhaps Harriet and I may even decide to spend some time at their clinic. We will need to check it out. I want now to concentrate and focus on a programme of exercise, meditation and visualization of the cancer I have and of my recovery from it. Other parts of the programme will continue to unfold just as they have so far. Meanwhile, I am resolved to do all that I can to gain the victory, to overcome.

Postscript — Growing in Grace

July 16, 1993
Teaneck, NJ

Today's first task was to edit my sermon on Habakkuk, "Faith in Spite of Everything", for inclusion in this volume as an appendix. For many years Habakkuk had been one of my favourite biblical books — "an old friend" I called him in Chapter 2. As an itinerant preacher I had delivered the sermon at least half a dozen times over the previous twenty years, modifying and refining it each time. As recently as December 6 last year — the second Sunday of Advent — I had revised and delivered it at Glen Rock. Editing it one more time I thought would be a breeze.

Anything but! In fact, I found that I couldn't use it at all. Habakkuk, it seemed, had taken two steps of faith, whereas three were necessary. His message needed to be augmented with a third step from the revelation in Jesus Christ. That is of course always a good interpretative principle for preachers of the Christian gospel using texts from the Hebrew Bible. In this case, however, it took me by surprise because of the power and clarity of Habakkuk's closing vision, which I will quote a bit later on.

Readers of Habakkuk's short book may remember that the first two chapters disclose a prophet dismayed with the corruption in Israel and even more dismayed that God would use the even more corrupt Chaldeans to punish the chosen people. He concluded this section with a mute, almost fatalistic acceptance of God's will expressed in words that are perhaps most familiar from their use at the opening of many worship services: "But the Lord is in his holy temple; let all the earth keep silence before Him!"

Many years later Habakkuk (some critics say a later author) added a third chapter, in which he more or less says to God, "OK, I accept your promise of deliverance, but please do it now." God responds with a majestic vision of God's glory and power which in turn prompts from Habakkuk one of the most beautiful lyric statements of faith to be found in any religious literature.

> Though the fig tree does not blossom,
> and no fruit is on the vines;
> though the produce of the olive fails
> and the fields yield no food;
> though the flock is cut off from the fold
> and there is no herd in the stalls,
> yet I will rejoice in the Lord;
> I will exult in the God of my salvation.
> God, the Lord, is my strength;
> he makes my feet like the feet of a deer,
> and makes me tread upon the heights.

Earlier that had been enough for me, as it was for Habakkuk. Indeed I had exulted in it with him. But now, as readers of Chapter 4 will recognize, I have discovered something more. I have discovered at a new depth that the God for whom I wait and watch, waits and watches with me — not only high and lifted up, but also alongside me in my suffering.

Discovering that an old sermon is unusable is of course a common experience for preachers. (If it isn't, it should be!) But not in this way. Not with a sermon lived by and repeatedly preached over twenty years, most recently with great feeling and conviction only a few months earlier. To me it was a powerful experience of growth even in the face of death, perhaps because it was in the face of death.

I was helped by that experience of growth related to faith to uncover another experience of growth I am having, this one related to hope. These days I hold out very little hope for my cancer to be cured. I haven't given up, but the statistics steadily weigh ever more heavily against it. In spite of that, I find my feelings of hope undiminished. How do I explain this even within the household of faith, to say nothing of a skeptical world? How do I keep people from feeling as they read this that I am clutching at a straw, deceiving myself, using hope as a form of escapism from the harsh reality of terminal illness and death? How do I communicate that in truth we do not sorrow as those who have no hope (1 Thessalonians 4:13)?

What is this hope, that abides in spite of everything? What forms does it take? I'm still discovering that, but I have a few initial answers. At a minimum, I know that the loved ones I leave behind will still be in touch with me, just as I have been for years with those who have passed over before me. Furthermore, I believe that my passing over is an entry into some form of life more rich and full than the one I have known. I believe that death is not the end, not the last word.

Having believed all this for many years, my feelings of hope are strong. I am not filled with dismay or anger or bitterness. This is true despite the aching disappointment I feel related to the people I want to be with and the things I would like to do in this life: the years of retirement with Harriet, increased availability to family and friends and the ecumenical experiment described in Chapter 9 — all of which now seem extremely unlikely.

To me, this experience of hope in spite of everything is even more important than the experience of faith in spite of everything. However mysterious, I know them to be real and am profoundly grateful for both.

There is of course a third word in the apostle's famous trilogy: of faith, hope, and *love*. In love, too, there is growth in the face of death, not first of all in my love, but rather in my experience of the love of others for me, and then, secondarily, in my love, as I try to respond to theirs. From the beginning of this experience, I have been bathed in love. Those early outpourings of love gave me strength and courage in the measure I then needed it. As the disease intensified its grip on my body, it seems that the capacity to love of those around me has kept growing until now it has reached depths I have not before known, or at least not recognized.

I find being so deeply loved a profoundly humbling experience. First, because I know this is a love that far surpasses anything I could ever have earned, and secondly because I do not know, and am inclined to doubt, whether I would be capable of giving the measure of love I am receiving. That likelihood has certainly been increased by my disease, but I still wonder, and that too is deeply humbling.

I have learned much in these past months. I would of course have preferred to receive the learning without having to pay so high a price; but since the price is being exacted in any event, I am grateful for what I have learned and for this opportunity to share some of it. It helps to lend purpose even to this painful phase of my life.

Purpose, and a sense of mystery. I confess that among my images of my own death, growing in faith, hope and love — in grace — did not occupy very much of my thoughts. For that matter, death did not. So I am grateful to know that even this last earthly act can not only be overcome by grace, but can itself be a means of grace.

Appendix 1

"I Am the Way, the Truth and the Life"

Scripture Lessons: Easter Sunday
Colossians 3:1-4   April 11, 1993
Luke 24:13-43   The Community Church
                           Glen Rock, New Jersey

If we are being observed by intelligent life from another planet, I am sure they have long since concluded that Christmas is a far more important holiday than Easter. Because Christmas has been commercialized, it permeates our society in a way that Easter does not. But if we look at these two festivals from a theological point of view, I believe we need to say that Easter is the high point of the Christian year.

At Christmas we are celebrating the glorious fact of the coming into the world of Jesus Christ, of God made flesh. At Easter we need to gather up that event as well as the whole life and ministry of Jesus Christ as we try somehow to understand the climax and the culmination of that ministry.

For a preacher, Easter is by far the more challenging of the two festivals. A preacher can talk at Christmas about birth knowing that everyone in the congregation has some experience of it. There is thus a point of contact for understanding at least a part of the Christmas message. Everyone can relate to the baby Jesus. None of us has any experience whatsoever of a resurrection.

So how do we talk about a resurrection? A sermon seems a peculiarly inadequate instrument for trying to interpret the meaning of a resurrection. A piece of prose simply isn't adequate to enter into the meaning of this mystery that we call the resurrection of Jesus Christ. Perhaps it is a day for poetry. It is surely a day for music and for art. It is a day in which the human spirit stretches itself to its outermost limits to know as much as it can of the fullness of God.

Complicating our attempts to communicate at both Christmas and Easter is the special challenge that attendance is swelled by the presence of those who are sometimes called Christmas and Easter Christians. We "regulars" want to welcome you. We want also to invite you to be present on many other occasions while avoiding the sort of scolding invitation that might well have the opposite effect. Our challenge, my challenge, is rather to meet the particular need and interest that brings you here on this Easter Sunday morning.

I therefore read with great interest a recent article in the *New York Times* by the religion editor Peter Steinfels, entitled "A Case for the Rarely Religious". He suggests that people who come to church only on Christmas and Easter are not interested in religion just on those two days. There is a deep undercurrent in life which suggests an extra dimension, and this suggestion grows stronger at Christmas and Easter, leading us to church on those particular days to appreciate and celebrate it. It is that undercurrent, that mystical chord of memory, that I want to touch this morning.

Peter Steinfels relates the article to Protestants, Catholics and Jews. I found the Catholic story by far the most charming. A woman who had grown up in Mexico said she could no longer relate to the whole range of what had been a heady brew of medieval, mystical Roman Catholicism. She finds what she now needs at Christmas and Easter in an Episcopal church which a friend of hers describes as "Catholic Lite". That seems a way of saying that people are looking for the values of the faith in which they were nourished, but they want those values stated in terms they can relate to the questions they are asking today. That is the challenge I want to take up this morning.

Complicating this further is the fact that on Easter Sunday there are still some people who want one more "scientific", historical discussion of the particular nature of the body of the resurrected Christ. Yesterday I read in the conservative evangelical magazine *Christianity Today* that US evangelicals are once again caught up in a theological firestorm of debate over the nature of the resurrected body of Jesus, arguing about distinctions which they admit no one really understands. At the end of the debate they still need to say, "It's a mystery". I can't imagine how that sort of argument can strengthen anybody's faith, and there is nothing of that in this sermon.

The resurrection is not a scientific and historically demonstrable fact. It is an article of faith. "I believe in the resurrection of the body" is a statement of faith. The early Christians were as surprised and stunned and confused by it as many of us are still today.

Even though the resurrection of Jesus stands at the centre of our faith as it did for the early Christians, the four gospels tell us very little about it. There is just one chapter in Matthew, Mark and Luke and only two chapters in John. This morning I wanted you to hear that long passage from Luke's gospel, so that you could feel for yourselves the jumble of emotions that characterized people on that first Easter Sunday. Let me highlight a few of them:
— fear on the one hand and hope on the other;
— belief on the one hand and disbelief on the other;
— doubt on the one hand and amazement on the other;
— grief on the one hand and joy on the other;
— anxiety on the one hand and confidence on the other.

This year I read these stories for the first time in the New Revised Standard Version. One verse tucked away towards the end of the passage from Luke's gospel summarizes this all beautifully, I believe: "In their joy they were disbelieving and still wondering."

Every one of us, I think, comes to this Easter Sunday morning with a sense of joy. We come also with a sense of wonder, with a sense of awe and perhaps also with a sense of skepticism. What does it mean to talk about the resurrection? What does it mean to say "I believe in the resurrection of the body"? Can we really believe this article of faith? Like the early Christians, in our joy we may be "disbelieving and still wondering".

Did you notice what Jesus did in response to their concerns and questions? He didn't lead a discussion of the nature of his resurrection body. He didn't talk with them about what it meant for him to die and then to be awakened from the sleep of death. He said, "Do you have something to eat here?" And they gave him a piece of boiled fish. Jesus wanted to communicate that he who walked to Emmaus and who stood there in the upper room with them was the same Jesus who earlier had walked the dusty roads of Palestine with James and John and Peter and the other disciples. He wanted to demonstrate that the Jesus whom they had known was fully present with them now.

Isn't that what you want to know? Isn't that why we are here on Easter Sunday morning? Isn't that why we say, "I believe in the resurrection of our Lord Jesus Christ", because we are wanting to confess, wanting to believe, wanting to celebrate that God is truly present with us?

What does it mean that God is here for me? I think there is no better answer in the Scriptures to that question than the words of our Lord himself in John 14, a passage often read at Christian funerals as we pass from life through death into life. Jesus says, "I am the Way, the Truth, and the Life."

"*I am the Way*." In the life I have to give there is meaning and purpose. In the life I have to offer, there is an answer to the question, "Is my life going anywhere?"

"*I am the Truth*". In the life I have to offer there is an answer to your questions: Is this the right way? Does the way I am walking fit the facts? Can it help me to deal with life as it really is?

"*I am the Life*". Is there some way in which my life can be enriched and enlarged? When I feel the Spirit moving and I know that movement cannot be experienced only in physical terms, is there some way I can get in touch with the fullness of this life of the Spirit surging within me?

Jesus doesn't say, "Here is a new way to live your life." He says, "I am the Way." Life in Jesus Christ is not a host of rules and regulations. Just because you keep the Ten Commandments and you don't kill your neighbour or bear false witness against a neighbour, just because you don't steal, and don't covet, it doesn't mean you are a religious person. There may be certain moral aspects to your life, but Jesus says the whole law is summed up in this: "You will love the Lord your God with all your strength, with all your soul, and with all your mind, and your neighbour as yourself."

Do you hear the difference? The ethical code is a system of rules and regulations, but the Way of Jesus has to do with relationships. Three times Jesus said to Peter, "Peter, do you love me?" He did not say, "Have you kept the law?" Religion is a way of discovering the transcendent dimension of life, a way to know more than you could conceivably know if you were only a physical being, a way to get a taste of life as it might be, not just of life as it is.

Life as it might be is life lived in relationship — relationship with God and relationship with our fellow human beings. Look at me, says Jesus. I am the Way. Do you want to know what it means to be religious? Follow me. Do you want to know what it means to lead life to the full? Follow me.

Now, you may say, "But Jesus, following you is the way that led to the cross." Jesus says it is the way of love, and the way of love always leads to the cross. To pick up the cross is to pick up someone else's burden, and if you love, you cannot go through this life without picking up somebody else's burden.

Then what does it mean that such a life is life lived to the full? Life lived to the full does not mean that you shed the burden. It means that when you pick up someone else's burden you feel a surge of spirit and strength within you that makes that burden bearable. You find as you go along that it somehow enriches your life.

This is all part of that strange mystery of claiming, as the gospels do, that on the cross God was glorified. Not just when Jesus ascended into heaven, but on the cross. The glory of God, the unending, unspeakable, indescribable love of God came through Jesus on the cross so that people could say, "So this is who God is". This is what it means to see the glory of God.

When we pick up our crosses and follow in the footsteps of Jesus Christ, people can see a little trace of that glory in us. We feel it ourselves as well, as life begins to burn with meaning, with a sense of joy and power impossible to find in any other way. That is why Jesus Christ says, "I am the Way", the way to the fullness of life.

Jesus also says, "I am the Truth". Can you trust this gospel? Is this revolutionary life-style, this backwards-forwards, upside-down life-style to which Jesus calls us, really livable out in the world? Jesus says, "I am the Truth". This claim to truth is twofold. It means first of all that the life Jesus is offering is completely clear of any false appearances. There is no facade here. Walking along the way of life with Jesus Christ is not passing through a Potemkin village. This is for real. The claim to truth also means that this gospel is faithful, it is secure, it will last until the end.

If that seems strange to you, stop to think for a moment. We are all inclined to dismiss the dreamers — Martin Luther King, Jr, for example. People said, "How in the world can his dream be fulfilled? We have lived in a segregated society for a long time. So he marches and preaches, and so a few other people march and preach. The dogs and the bullwhips and the batons are going to win in the long run. We will live in a society separate and unequal forever. That's the way the world is."

Now look at the world. Look at it and ask: Who is the realist? Is the incredible devastation in our inner cities because of the dreams of Martin Luther King, Jr? Or because we didn't follow his dreams? Who is the realist?

King used to insist that the only way the world could really live would be for every man, woman, and child to live as a full-fledged member of what he called "the beloved community", a community in which everyone who is black could be fully human and fully black, in which everyone who is white could be fully human and fully white. Then we would live in a world where it is possible for all of us to live together. He was the realist. The dreamer was the realist. It was the dreamer who told the truth.

Or look at the arms race in which we have engaged over the last five decades. Were the realists the people who said the only way to protect ourselves is by Mutually Assured Destruction? Well, we have the mutual destruction. We have a world economy in ruins. We have Russia gasping for its life, still full of all kinds of danger. We can say the same thing about the environment and the economy. Who is the realist — the militarist or the peacemaker?

Sisters and brothers, the way of peace, justice, love is the only true way. Other things may appear to be true for a moment, but they are a mirage. They will fade away. The long visions are those rooted deep in human history, in the fundamental community values that human beings have established over the years. They are visions that dare to conserve what is true and to claim the promises of the gospel. They promise the beloved community, fullness of life to every person, they dream of a world in which no one has everything but everyone has enough.

I am the Truth. The way of love is the only way to walk in the world. It is the only way to life.

And so Jesus makes a third claim: I am the Life. God is often described in the Hebrew scriptures as the fountain of life. To be created in the image of God is to have within us a spring of life. To fulfill that image of God we need to use every means at our disposal — whether it's art or music or literature or dance or song or work or love — in some way to nurture and express those powerful feelings within us. Jesus says, I am the source of that life. In me you can experience its abundance. "I am come that you may have life and have it abundantly." "I am the Way, the Truth and the Life."

What does the resurrection have to do with all of this? The resurrection means that those surges of life we feel, those dreams of a better world to which we would love to cling but are not quite certain we dare, those times when we walk the way of life on behalf of someone else and feel our own lives renewed within us are not illusions but reality. When I say "I believe in the resurrection of the body", it means that those are the great realities of life and that all those other things I think are real may in fact be the mirages.

The apostle John puts it beautifully when he suggests that to come to life in Jesus Christ is to begin to experience the new life in a first resurrection. The life we receive in Jesus Christ is literally larger than life. It cannot be contained within our physical existence. It cannot be contained within history. It is literally something that bursts into our world from another world and needs to be fulfilled again in another world. It also means that those moments that we treasure and cherish in our lives are carried over from this world into another world, so that in the Book of Revelation this same apostle John can say that "the honour and glory of the nations" — everything that is beautiful and precious in life — will pass from this life into another life, and we can rejoice in it in that life.

I believe in the resurrection of the body. I believe that the most precious moments of reality that I experience in this life are not figments of my imagination. I believe they are gifts from God. I believe that they are gifts from our Lord, Jesus Christ. I believe that the resurrection of Jesus Christ is an eternal testimony that they will never pass away. And that no matter what happens, neither life nor death nor principalities nor powers nor any other thing in all creation can separate me from life. I believe in the resurrection of the body.

Appendix 2

"I Believe in the Communion of Saints"

Scripture lessons: All Saints Day
Psalm 84:1,2,10a,12   November 1, 1992
Hebrews 11:32-12:2a   The Community Church
John 14:1-3   Glen Rock, New Jersey

All Saints Day is the day on which we celebrate the presence of all the saints who are with us and who are in the presence of God. We confess our faith in that presence every time we repeat the Apostles' Creed: "I believe in the communion of saints."

The literal meaning of the word "saint", used often in the New Testament, is simply someone who is set apart into the presence of God. When Paul begins his letters, even to that extraordinarily troubled congregation in Corinth, he usually says, "called to be saints". We are all called to be saints.

In ordinary usage, however, we apply the word "saint" to people who convey a special sense of the presence of God. As Christians, we all long for that experience of the presence of God, so we quite naturally honour such people in the hope that some of their experience of God's presence in their lives will rub off on us as well. So we set the saints apart once again, not only from the world, but also from the church. We shouldn't. The calling belongs to us all.

This desire to honour those who are close to God led to all kinds of abuse in the medieval church. As the scriptures were not read or taught, as the presence of God disappeared into remote obfuscations, as darkness displaced light, people wanted something they could hang onto, someone they could touch so that they could feel themselves to be in the presence of God. Over time, as faith gave way to superstition, they began to pray to the saints, endowing them with all sorts of magical powers.

All Saints Eve (also called Hallowed Eve and now sec-
ularized to Halloween) originated as a joyful celebration
of the presence with us of those saints who are also fully
present with God. Church authorities gradually cast this
festival in a judgmental mode and made it an instrument
for priestly and hierarchical control of the church by
inciting fear and trepidation among the people.

The Reformation quite naturally led to an overreaction
against the overreaction. Many of its leaders said that
because the role of the saints had been so terribly dis-
torted, the reformation of the church required removing
from the churches all the statues of the saints so that
people would not be tempted to pray to them. The idea of
All Saints Day was more or less eradicated. As a result,
we lost a sense of the fullness of the communion of saints.
We lost a sense of the presence with us of those who are
now fully in the presence of God.

Deep down most of us feel some intimation of this
relationship. Moreover, a little while ago as we sang that
great hymn of the church, "The Church's One Foundation", we spoke the words:

The Church on earth hath union
with God, the three in one,
and mystic sweet communion
with those whose rest is won.

This is by no means a little romanticism and sentimen-
talism left over from another era which doesn't fit in our
rational, enlightened age. It points rather to the fullness of
the communion of saints of which we here together even
in our highest moments have only a preliminary foretaste.

"Communion" is another one of the great words of the
New Testament. The Greek word which it translates is
koinonia, a word we have taken over into English, using

it, for example, to describe "koinonia groups", a usage drawn largely from the Book of Acts, where we read of the Christians being together and having fellowship or communion — *koinonia*.

What creates such communion? Well, first of all we are united by need. No doubt that need takes different forms for each of us. Sometimes our need takes the form of guilt or shame or despair, from which we want to be released. Perhaps our need is only to be in relationship with other people. Maybe we want to share in service with other people, because we know that when we put our hands together towards a common task, our hearts are also bonded together. A fellowship develops among us, a bond, a communion; and we find ourselves tied closely with the other people with whom we share that common task. Common work builds communion, common life. Underlying the communion that springs from common work, we intuitively sense a community of being in which we share not only our skills and abilities but our persons, our selves.

In the church, this communion of being takes on several extra dimensions. It is not only communion with one another's beings, but with God as well, the common source of all our beings. Because we belong to God in Christ, we all belong to each other in a bond that can never be equaled by a merely two-dimensional relationship of person to person. There is in the church a third dimension, and perhaps even a fourth, since we are bound together not only with one another and with God but also with the whole Christian community through all time and in every place. When we are baptized we are not just baptized into a local congregation but into the whole church of Christ from the Year One to the Year Whenever. And when we die, our bodies are returned to the earth and to its Creator, as we are drawn into the presence of God and the presence of the saints through all the ages.

The Orthodox churches, who have so much enriched my understanding of what it means to be a Christian, emphasize that this communion is rooted in the very nature of God. Father, Son and Holy Spirit exist as separate persons to be sure, but within the community of the Trinity. All Christians believe that of course, but the Orthodox have helped us to recapture and to deepen the importance of this doctrine for our common life.

I am personally persuaded that for the forty or seventy years in which Orthodox Christians in Central and Eastern Europe lived under the tyranny of communism, no small part of their ability to sustain their existence as persons in the face of an oppressive social system was that this communion in the Trinity stood at the very heart of their faith. They could see that although God is one, yet God is also three. Just as community cannot be sacrificed to individualism, so personhood cannot be sacrificed to communalism. Personal self-identity cannot be eradicated by any communalism, however powerful.

The Orthodox, together with the Roman Catholics and to some extent Lutherans, Episcopalians, Moravians and Swedenborgians, are generally more aware than we in the Reformed tradition that this communion of the saints includes the heavenly community. The author of the Hebrews speaks of our being surrounded by "a great cloud of witnesses". He is speaking of all those whose rest is won. We live in the presence of those who are fully in the presence of God.

I want to celebrate this sound biblical doctrine by sharing some of my own experiences of it. I remember very vividly, for example, the day my father died some fifteen years ago. I was in my office in New York one evening, working late, when the telephone call came. To my surprise I didn't cry — and seemingly couldn't cry. So I began to make preparations for our family's travel to Minnesota where the funeral would be conducted, all the while wanting to get in touch with my feelings.

Forty-five minutes later I was driving up Riverside Drive, headed for the George Washington Bridge, thinking about my father and wondering why in the world I couldn't get in touch with all that I was feeling. Then I recalled that I often used to sing the second verse of the old favourite gospel song, "When the Saints Go Marching In" with him in mind:

> My father loved the Savior,
> what a soldier he had been,
> but his steps will be more steady
> when the saints go marching in.

Suddenly my father was present to me, and I began to cry. I had found a channel for my grief and bereavement, a channel that could handle it — and that I could handle. In the fifteen years since then, every time I hear that verse or I think of it, it is one of the many ways in which my father is present to me.

Two years later my mother also passed over. From her I learned the Dutch language, mostly through singing the Psalms in her native tongue. We used to sing them together from a little book which she called her "*Psalm-boekje*". Her favourite was that great lament of Reformed Dutch pietism, Psalm 42:

> As the deer longs for flowing streams,
> so my soul longs for you, O God.

The Dutch Reformed sang that psalm again and again, and so did she and I. When I want to experience her particular presence I often take her little psalm book off the shelf and sing again the words " '*t Hijgend hert de jacht ontkomen...*".

Many of you surely have your own symbols of being in touch with those who have passed over. But it is not always so easy as I have just portrayed it. Sometimes there are barriers in the way. I remember some time ago being in a group in which the leader said that if any of us was feeling separated from someone to whom we could not relate because that person was no longer alive, he or she could ask any other group member to represent that particular person. "Go to them," he said, "and tell them what's standing between you and them and ask them to forgive you." The young woman sitting next to me stood up, turned to me and said, "Would you be my father?" I said, "Of course I will." Crying, she said, "I want to say to you, Dad, that I didn't mean those terrible things I said to you on the day you died. I didn't mean them." I could say to her, "I know you didn't, Sally. I know you didn't mean them. They're troubling to you, but they're not troubling to me because I've passed over and I've left all that behind."

Some of you know that I had a brother killed in Korea in the early 1950s. I was just a boy, and like many brothers we sometimes had our misunderstandings. At the time he went off to war, we were in the middle of such a minor misunderstanding; and we were too stupid and too young to know how to fix it. We both wanted to before he went off to war but neither of us knew how — and of course he never came back. I struggled for years with the fact that we had not made things right before he died. A few years ago I went to visit North and then South Korea. Through friends I had found out exactly the place where my brother had died, only to discover that it was in the demilitarized zone, so I couldn't actually go to the very place. I could and did look at it through field glasses, and I could and did talk to representatives of the North Korean government. In that presence and in that place, what had happened thirty-five years ago came rushing back into me with a power that I didn't know could possibly be true any longer. I stood there then and wept in the strong arms of a friend. I recalled that experience again this week. And suddenly, in juxtaposition with the story I just told about the group I was in, I realized that I no longer had to ask my brother for forgiveness. We were in communion, because I had gotten rid of that particular barrier.

What has all of this to do with the communion of the saints? It is important to recognize that those who are gathered into the presence of God are free of all pain. The promise is fulfilled. They are free. If there is any barrier between us and anyone who has passed over, the barrier is within us. They have transcended it. So can we.

I believe in the communion of saints because I belong to God, and my loved ones who have passed over belong to God, and because you belong to God, and because everyone who believes in Jesus Christ belongs to God. We belong to one another. This is the way the apostle Paul puts it in that magnificent statement of faith at the end of Romans 8:

> Who will separate us from the love of Christ? Will hardship, or distress, or persecution, or famine, or nakedness, or peril, or sword? No, in all these things we are more than conquerors through him who loved us. For I am persuaded that neither death, nor life, nor angels, nor principalities, nor powers, nor things present, nor things to come, nor height, nor depth, nor anything else in all creation, will be able to separate us from the love of God in Christ Jesus our Lord.

I believe in the communion of saints.

Some Notes on
Ecumenical Immobility

In Chapter 9, I stated that I do not think the churches will respond to the call for a new ecumenical vision "for several simple but powerful reasons" which I promised to elaborate in this appendix.

First, the main instruments of the ecumenical movement, the councils of churches, are now almost completely captive to the churches. Almost totally eroded is both the understanding of the councils as agents of the ecumenical movement and their capacity in that role to stand over against the churches when that becomes necessary. Instead they are seen almost exclusively as agents of the churches and subject to their control. Ernst Lange made that point already in the 1970s in his book *And Yet It Moves* — still, I think, the best overall book on the present state of the ecumenical movement. In the twenty years since the publication of his book, the control of the churches has been even more firmly locked into place, just as he assumed it would be.

With the churches in control, it follows that most of the leading participants in most council meetings are either ecclesiastical bureaucrats or hierarchs, who are mostly prisoners of their positions. Real movement toward unity would render most of their present positions redundant. Few of them seem to see that it would also create many much more exciting positions. Nor do they seem to see that, at least in the US, the denominations are dying and that their positions are disappearing anyway. Very few bureaucrats, church bureaucrats included, are willing to put their positions at risk — even in the face of open violation of truth or justice, much less for the sake of a vision only dimly perceived.

Each of these two facts, church control and the bureaucratic and hierarchical domination of council meetings which enforces it, is supported by its own increasingly powerful ideology. First, the ideology of church control. In point of fact, none of the churches can actually lay claim to being a church in the classic understanding of a community offering up to God the fruits of a whole culture of a whole people of a given region. To be sure, the most vigorous claimants of the word "church", the Orthodox and the Roman Catholic, come closest to this. But even they fall short. Nowhere is this more evident than in the salad-bowl society of the United States. Amidst the melange of religions in America, Roman Catholics have long since had to admit that they are one denomination among many. During the last decade, the Orthodox, too, have openly confessed that their inability to solve the jurisdictional problem and create one Orthodox Church in the USA in effect reduces them to denominations as well. The Orthodox understand that one cannot have more than one church in any one place at the same time.

Yet, rather than integrating these new facts into a renewed ecclesiology which could be a powerful instrument for the fuller manifestation of the church, one, holy, catholic and apostolic, the Protestant denominations, at least at the national level, are increasingly asserting their "churchliness". They have failed to recognize that the traditional Orthodox and Roman Catholic ecclesiologies which claim the status of church no longer fit the facts. Instead the Protestant denominations have more and more appropriated that outdated ecclesiology for themselves, especially in their attitudes toward the councils.

They need not assert that ecclesiology vis-a-vis other churches since other churches no longer constitute a real threat to the continuing separate existence of any denomination. The ecumenical movement does, particularly in its conciliar form. The ecclesiology of denominational churchliness serves as a bulwark against that threat. Claiming such churchliness for themselves alone, the denominations continue to deny to the councils and other instruments of unity the ecclesial significance that would empower them to challenge the continuing separate existence of the denominations. This is done in the face of all ecumenical experience which testifies to such ecclesial significance. Is there anyone who has not recognized in an ecumenical service of worship a fuller presence of God than is possible in their denominational isolation? That is a sign of ecclesial significance.

Closely related to this ideology of denominational churchliness is the ideology of pluralism, which serves to lock into place the phenomenon of plurality and give it priority over unity. This ideology is a bulwark against the threat of finding essential unity amidst our rich diversity. It too serves to nullify the ecumenical movement. Plurality is a cultural phenomenon which in its various manifestations can be integrated in an historical process. Pluralism, however, is an ideology that by definition claims to stand outside of such historical processes. The effect is to place plurality beyond the range of human action, thus serving to assure the churches of the legitimacy of their continuing separate existence, the hierarchies of their perpetuation and the bureaucrats of their positions.

Perhaps it is necessary to say here that I would not want my objections to the ideology of pluralism to be understood as implying endorsement of the present concern for "limits to diversity". On the contrary, I believe that intentional (and not merely accidental) interaction of diversity is the way to unity. Consequently I believe that the "limits to diversity" approach to ecumenical issues is rooted in an error of methodology so serious that it precludes the possibility of reaching a fruitful resolution of our differences.

The methodological error is that concern about the "limits to diversity" addresses the various responses to our differences at the circumference, at the outer "limits" of acceptability. A more fruitful methodology would keep the focus on the questions and their connection to the centre.

In other words, instead of asking whether a certain theological formulation is within the boundaries of the tradition, we should ask whether the questions being raised (which are almost always already on the boundaries) are being pursued in the spirit of the Tradition as revealed in Jesus Christ, who is the centre. Any response to the questions which is arrived at under such a guidance of that Spirit will by definition be within the Tradition. To be sure, it may stretch the boundaries of the tradition, but that is essential to its continuing power and relevance (see Acts 15).

Clearly the approach I am advocating places great emphasis on our need to "test the spirits" (1 John 4:1-6) for the present presence of the Spirit in the search here and now rather than relying primarily on testing the results of the search against the Spirit's earlier witness there and then when we, like the disciples of old, may not have been prepared to receive this new teaching of the Spirit (John 16:12ff.). This methodology is, I believe, faithful to the well-known affirmation of Georges Florovsky that

> loyalty to tradition means not only concord with the past, but in a certain sense freedom from the past... Tradition is the constant abiding of the spirit, and not only the memory of words. Tradition is a charismatic, not an historical principle (*Bible, Church, Tradition*, Vol. 1, p. 80).

Focusing on the centre suggests, even invites, the growth of the Tradition; focusing on the "limits of diversity" encourages its stagnation and ossification by making Tradition an "historical principle".

Unfortunately all I am able to do here is to identify the issue. I have neither time, energy nor space to develop it further.*

The two institutional factors mentioned above, church control of the ecumenical movement and bureaucrats and hierarchs as prisoners of their position, together with the ideologies of denominational churchliness and supra-historical pluralism, are obstacles which seem to me too powerful to overcome in the present institutional framework. Indeed, this observation seems indisputable in the light of at least fifty years of history clearly demonstrated in the WCC and in the NCC in the United States as well as in most other places. Change I believe is possible only if the systems within the ecumenical movement themselves undergo radical change. That change is the movement from below which I have sketched at the end of Chapter 9.

The fruits of such a movement from below would of course be much more easily realized if the denominations themselves would make it happen. However difficult this would be politically, procedurally it would be a simple matter for them to do so. For example, instead of the present limping offices of worship in most denominations, an office of ecumenical worship could be created, with the

---

* Those who are interested can see the problem of "limits of diversity" clearly reflected in the symposium on "Owning the Spirit" in the July 15, 1991 *Christianity and Crisis*. Of particular interest are the contributions of John Deschner and Leonid Kishkovsky, both for their content and because both have been leading participants in Faith and Order discussions for many years.

staff of the denominations seconded to it and thereby
made accountable to the NCC. This would be in sharp
contrast to — and much more fruitful than — the present
system of bringing the denominational staff together from
time to time in an ecumenical setting.

Such an action however would require a recognition
by the denominations that ecumenical worship, rather than
denominational worship, is the wave of the future, not just
because it is inevitable in some quarters, but because it is
faithful to the Tradition, the integrity of the church,
service to the people and capacity to show forth the
fulness of God's glory. Such recognition cannot be
achievable by a denomination as a whole, either in worship or in most other areas of congregational life. On the
other hand, some congregations in all denominations I
believe would seize the opportunity. The challenge I think
is to bring them together in a movement.